D0220451

CONTENTS

PREFACE

Unlike other textbooks of laboratory medicine, this fourth edition of *A Guide to Laboratory Investigations* is written by a full-time practising general practitioner familiar with the daily challenges of interpreting an increasing number and variety of laboratory tests. This new edition has updates on long established and familiar tests as well as interpretations of newer tests such as PSA velocity and free/total PSA and coeliac serology. There are also several new guidelines on appropriate investigations in specific clinical conditions such as appropriate laboratory investigations in heart failure, investigations in the management of female infertility, specific lipid monitoring in diabetes and guidance on the appropriate use of MSUs in suspected UTIs (are MSUs always really necessary?). There are also guidelines for monitoring renal function in patients on ACE inhibitors, monitoring statin therapy and guidelines on testing patients on disease modifying anti-rheumatic drugs: what to test and when to stop such drugs.

Completely new interpretations of hospital-based tests include interpretation of Doppler scans in the management of leg ulcers and interpreting DEXA scans in screening for osteoporosis.

General practitioners continue to depend upon and utilise laboratory investigations to the maximum and the rapidly changing technology and interpretation of results continues to be well served by this authoritative text. Hospital doctors and practice nurses will also continue to find *A Guide to Laboratory Investigations* an invaluable daily reference.

Michael McGhee
March 2003

GLOSSARY

ACE	angiotensin-converting enzyme
AIDS	acquired immune deficiency syndrome
ALO	*Actinomyces*-like organisms
ALT	alanine transferase
ANA	antinuclear antibody
ANCA	antineutrophil cytoplasmic antibody
APC-R	activated protein C resistance
ASO	antistreptoylsin-O
AST	aspartate transferase
BMI	body mass index
BP	blood pressure
BPH	benign prostatic hypertrophy
CABG	coronary artery bypass graft
CAD	coronary artery disease
CCDC	Consultant in Communicable Disease Control
CCF	congestive cardiac failure
CEA	carcino-embryonic antigen
CHD	coronary heart disease
CIN	cervical intra-epithelial neoplasia
CK	creatine kinase
CLL	chronic lymphatic leukaemia
CMV	cytomegalovirus
CREST	calcinosis, Raynaud's, oesophageal hypermobility, sclerodactyly, telangiectasia
CRP	C-reactive protein
CSF	cerebrospinal fluid
CVA	cerebrovascular accident
DEXA	dual energy X-ray absorptiometry
DIC	disseminated intravascular coagulation
DNA	deoxyribonucleic acid

DVT	deep vein thrombosis
EBV	Epstein–Barr virus
ECG	electrocardiograph
EDTA	ethylenediamine tetra-acetic acid
ELISA	enzyme-linked immunosorbent assay
ESR	erythrocyte sedimentation rate
FAI	free androgen index
FDP	fibrin degradation products
FSH	follicle-stimulating hormone
FT_4I	free thyroxine index
GBM	glomerular basement membrane
GFR	glomerular filtration rate
GGT	gamma-glutamyl transferase
GTT	glucose tolerance test
Hb	haemoglobin
HbA_1	haemoglobin alpha-1
HCG	human chorionic gonadotrophin
HCl	hydrochloric acid
HDL	high-density lipoprotein
HDLC	high-density-lipoprotein cholesterol
HDN	haemolytic disease of the newborn
5HIAA	5-hydroxyindole acetic acid
HLA	human leucocyte antigen
HPV	human papilloma virus
HVA	homovanillic acid
HVS	high vaginal swab
IDDM	insulin-dependent diabetes mellitus
IHD	ischaemic heart disease
INR	international normalised ratio
IUCD	intrauterine contraceptive device
KCCT	kaolin cephalin clotting time
LATS	long-acting thyroid stimulator
LDH	lactic dehydrogenase
LDL	low-density lipoprotein
LDLC	low-density-lipoprotein cholesterol
LE	lupus erythematosus
LFT	liver function test
LH	luteinising hormone
LUC	large unstained cells
MAOI	monoamine oxidase inhibitor

MCV	mean corpuscular volume
MDS	myelodysplastic syndrome
MI	myocardial infarction
MSU	midstream urine specimen
NIDDM	non-insulin-dependent diabetes mellitus
NSAID	non-steroidal anti-inflammatory drug
OA	osteoarthritis
OTC	over the counter
PA	pernicious anaemia
PCV	packed cell volume
PE	pulmonary embolism
PID	pelvic inflammatory disease
PRV	polycythaemia rubra vera
PSA	prostate-specific antigen
PUO	pyrexia of unknown origin
PVD	peripheral vascular disease
RA	rheumatoid arthritis
RAHA	rheumatoid arthritis haemagglutination assay
RBC	red blood cell count
SBE	subacute bacterial endocarditis
SCD	sickle-cell disease
SGOT	serum glutamic oxaloacetic transaminase
SGPT	serum glutamic pyruvic transaminase
SHBG	sex-hormone-binding globulin
SLE	systemic lupus erythematosus
T_3	tri-iodothyronine
T_4	thyroxine
TB	tuberculosis
TBG	thyroxine-binding globulin
TC	total cholesterol
TFT	thyroid function test
TG	triglyceride
TIA	transient ischaemic attack
TIBC	total iron-binding capacity
TOP	termination of pregnancy
TPHA	*Treponema pallidum* haemagglutination assay
TPO	thyroid peroxidase
TRAb	thyrotrophin antibody
TRH	thyrotrophin-releasing hormone
TSH	thyroid-stimulating hormone

UTI	urinary tract infection
VDRL	Venereal Disease Reference Laboratory
VLDL	very-low-density lipoprotein
VMA	vanillylmandelic acid
WBC	white blood cell count
WCC	white cell count
Ca^{2+}	calcium
Cl^-	chloride
Cu^{2+}	copper
dl	decilitre
fl	femtolitre
g	gram
H_2O	water
IM	intramuscular
IU	international unit
IV	intravenous
K^+	potassium
kU	kilo-unit
l	litre
Li^+	lithium
mEq	milli-equivalent
Mg^{2+}	magnesium
mg	milligram
μg	microgram
μmol	micromole
mIU	milli-international unit
ml	millilitre
mm	millimetre
mmHg	millimetres of mercury pressure
mmol	millimole
mU	milli-unit
Na^+	sodium
ng	nanogram
nmol	nanomole
pg	picogram
pmol	picomole
U	unit
Zn^{2+}	zinc

%	percentage	<	less than	=	equals
>	more than	≥	more than or equal to		

INTRODUCTION

Consultation and referral

General practitioners vary in their use of the laboratory services, with variation of up to 10-fold between comparable practices in the rates of blood tests requested per patient. Variation occurs not only in the use of the pathology and radiology facilities, but also in the use of specialist referral.

Although many investigations are performed in order to confirm or refute a clinical suspicion (e.g. anaemia or hypothyroidism), an increasing number of tests are conducted as part of screening (e.g. Well Man and Well Woman screening clinics). Because investigations are used in this way, and as reports contain more information than is requested, unexpected findings (e.g. mild thrombocytopenia) are not uncommon.

The GP then has to decide whether to react to the test or ignore it, if it is not significantly outside the normal range. Whilst many laboratories publish a guide to their own local laboratory values, which may vary according to the technique employed by the laboratory, it is left to the clinician who is requesting the test to decide on appropriate action as a result of the test.

The intention of this desktop ready reference is to help practitioners to make a more informed choice with regard to further investigation or referral as appropriate, and to prompt further investigations if they would be helpful. There will never be any substitute for a good clinical history and thorough physical examination, but this book will hopefully fill in some of the blanks when an appropriate history, examination and investigations have taken place.

HAEMATOLOGY

Referring to a haematologist

Clinical haematology, as practised in the UK, differs from most other medical specialities in one very important aspect. The haematologist who is asked to see a patient not only takes the history and examines the patient but also, having decided on the appropriate investigations, will then usually perform the key tests (e.g. bone-marrow biopsy), examine the material and make the diagnosis. He or she will then prescribe the treatment and perform the follow-up of the patient.

Almost all health districts offer a laboratory and clinical service. Many of the investigations and treatments are conducted on a day-patient basis. Sometimes the hospital performs the test and the patient's GP is asked to monitor and adjust the dose of certain drugs (e.g. warfarin and second-line antirheumatic drugs).

Near patient testing, particularly international normalised ratio (INR) testing (*see* p. 29) is already practised in some countries and may soon be used in the UK.

Cases that the haematologist must see

There are a number of haematological conditions that must be referred to a consultant.

HAEMATOLOGICAL MALIGNANCIES

Acute leukaemia

Few doctors would argue against the urgent referral of any patient with suspected acute leukaemia reported on a blood film. The exact diagnosis can only be made using a microscope, and as the diagnosis determines the treatment offered, and patients who are well at presentation do better than patients who present in a crisis, early referral is obligatory.

The following unexpected haematological findings *should be referred immediately*.

- Abnormal blood films, such as abnormal, immature or odd-shaped cells, are always commented on by the haematologist, who will usually indicate that referral is necessary.
- Lymphocytosis $>15 \times 10^9/l$.
- Refractory anaemia (i.e. anaemia which fails to respond to haematinics).
- Obscure anaemias (e.g. those where the blood film carries a comment such as 'spherocytes seen').
- Haemoglobinopathies and thalassaemias. Remember that an unexplained hypochromic microcytic anaemia may well represent thalassaemia and not iron deficiency.
- Suspected bleeding disorders such as clotting defects.

Red cell indices

HAEMOGLOBIN (Hb)

In an individual the haemoglobin level remains fairly constant, but between individuals there may be variation of up to 3 g/dl.

- A reduction in plasma volume caused by dehydration or strenuous muscular exercise may increase the haemoglobin by up to 1.5 g/dl.

- A 5–10% drop in haemoglobin may be seen on assuming a lying position from standing.
- Normal range (g/dl) for adults:
  male, 13.5–18
  female, 11.5–16.5.
- Normal range (g/dl) for children:
  at birth, 16.5 (13.5–19.5)
  2 weeks, 16.5 (12.5–20.5)
  2 months, 11.5 (9–14)
  6 months, 11.5 (9.5–13.5)
  puberty (male), 13–16
  puberty (female), 12–16.

Abnormal test results

- Raised Hb suggests:
  polycythaemia (*see* below)
  smoking (increases the Hb due to increased carboxyhaemoglobin)
  hypoxia and some renal conditions in which excess erythropoietin is produced.

Smoking increases the haemoglobin level in direct proportion to the number of cigarettes smoked.

- Lowered Hb indicates anaemia. In young females the most common cause is heavy menstrual loss. Other red cell indices can help to identify the likely cause of anaemia. Clinical symptoms of anaemia often do not appear until the haemoglobin level has fallen to 7–9 g/dl.

RED CELL COUNT

Male, $4.0–5.9 \times 10^{12}/l$
Female, $3.8–5.2 \times 10^{12}/l$

- High RBC counts seen in polycythaemia and in dehydration.
- Low RBC counts seen in any cause of anaemia and thalassaemia.

HAEMATOCRIT OR PACKED CELL VOLUME (PCV)

- Normal range (ml) for adults:
    male, 0.40–0.54 (41–54%)
    female, 0.35–0.47 (35–47%).

- Normal range (ml) for children:
    at birth, 0.42–0.54
    1–3 years, 0.29–0.4
    4–10 years, 0.36–0.38.

- Raised levels indicate increased red blood cell production (e.g. chronic hypoxia associated with pulmonary disease and congenital heart disease, polycythaemia rubra vera (PRV) or lowered plasma volume (e.g. dehydration, stress polycythaemia or pseudopolycythaemia).

- Lowered PCV is found in acute blood volume loss, anaemia and overhydration.

- PCV of >0.45 is strongly associated with thrombo-embolic disease.

- PCV of >0.52 should always be investigated.

POLYCYTHAEMIA

- PCV of >0.48 in females.

- PCV of >0.51 in males.

- Hypertension, smoking and stress can cause stress polycythaemia or pseudopolycythaemia.

- In primary polycythaemia (previously know as polycythaemia rubra vera) Hb is raised, haematocrit or PCV is raised and RBC is raised.

- In polycythaemia rubra vera, as well as the red cell changes, the white cell count and platelet count are also raised.

- Pseudopolycythaemia or stress polycythaemia is characterised by a raised haemoglobin level, a normal white cell count, normal platelet count, normal red cell mass and decreased plasma volume.

- Up to 15% of patients with PRV will eventually develop a form of leukaemia which is often resistant to chemotherapy.

MEAN CORPUSCULAR VOLUME (MCV)

- Normal range (fl) is 80–99, although it is lower in children (78 at age 1 year). The mean cell volume increases with age in males.

Abnormal test results

- Raised MCV suggests:
  vitamin B_{12} or folate deficiency (either dietary or due to malabsorption)
  myxoedema
  alcohol or liver disease
  occasionally aplastic anaemia and myelodysplasias
  haemolysis
  aplasia or marrow infiltration.
- Vitamin B_{12} and/or folate deficiency both cause a raised MCV, usually accompanied by a low Hb, low white cell count and low platelets.
- After 3 months (the lifespan of the RBC) the MCV should return to normal, failure to do so warrants further investigation, e.g. thyroid function tests or bone-marrow examination for myelodysplasia.
- Checking the reticulocyte count after commencing B_{12} or folate replacement confirms new red blood cell production in response to treatment.
- Lowered MCV (microcytosis) suggests:
  chronic blood loss, commonly menstrual in young females or occult blood loss due to gastrointestinal disease in older patients
  iron-deficiency anaemia
  thalassaemia
  sideroblastic anaemia (myelodysplastic syndrome)
  anaemia of chronic disease.

- Microcytosis, especially in the absence of anaemia, is strongly suggestive of the thalassaemia trait, especially in patients of foreign origin. Electrophoresis will usually show a raised HbA$_2$ unless there is a coexisting iron deficiency.

- The MCV may be normal in anaemia of chronic disease, uraemia, acute blood loss, myeloproliferative disorders and bone-marrow infiltration, or where vitamin B$_{12}$ or folate deficiency are combined with iron deficiency or thalassaemia.

MEAN CORPUSCULAR HAEMOGLOBIN (MCH)

- Normal range (pg) is 27–33.

- The MCH and mean corpuscular haemoglobin concentration (MCHC) should not be interpreted alone but in conjunction with the other red cell parameters.

Abnormal test results

- Raised MCH suggests:
  vitamin B$_{12}$ or folate deficiency
  myxoedema.

- Lowered MCH suggests:
  iron deficiency
  thalassaemia
  chronic blood loss
  megaloblastic anaemia.

MEAN CORPUSCULAR HAEMOGLOBIN CONCENTRATION (MCHC)

- Normal range (g/dl) is 32–36.

Abnormal test results

- Lowered MCHC suggests:
  iron deficiency
  blood loss.

- Raised MCHC may be seen in the presence of spherocytes and sickle cells.

ACTIVATED PROTEIN C RESISTANCE (APC-R)

- Activated protein C resistance is an inherited condition characterised by factor V being abnormally resistant to degradation by activated protein C, resulting in a tendency for blood to clot more easily.

- The gene responsible for APC-R was discovered in 1994 in Leiden, The Netherlands, and is often called factor V Leiden.

- APC-R is probably the commonest inherited condition known, affecting 5–8% of the population.

- Anyone with APC-R has a 50% chance of a brother or sister having it, and will have one parent who has it.

- Some patients may have a double dose of APC-R, if both parents have the gene, and are therefore at even greater risk of blood clots.

- The normal range of APC resistance is 2.2–7.0.

Abnormal test results

A low test result indicates a higher-than-normal likelihood of thrombosis. High-oestrogen oral contraceptive pills should be avoided. Prophylaxis against thrombosis may be considered in major surgery.

ANTI-CARDIOLIPIN IgG

Anti-cardiolipin IgG is an antibody against the beta-2 glycoprotein coagulation system. A significantly raised level is indicative of an increased risk of thrombosis, and is often found in autoimmune disease and in patients with recurrent miscarriages (more than three), and is thought to be due to placental thrombosis.

- The results for levels of cardiolipin antibodies should be interpreted with caution.

- Low positive levels may be found in normal people.
- Interpretive guidelines:
  normal, ≤7.2 U/ml
  negative, <13.3
  low positive, 13.4–19.9
  moderate, 20–80
  high, >80.1.

Anaemia

COMMON CAUSES OF ANAEMIA

Anaemia with decreased MCV

This may be due to:
  iron deficiency
  thalassaemia and some haemoglobinopathies
  anaemia of chronic disease.

- Further investigations:
  blood film;
  serum ferritin (the most useful test for iron deficiency)
  electrophoresis
  reticulocyte count
  faecal occult blood.

Anaemia with normal MCV

This may be due to:
  acute blood loss
  haemolysis
  anaemia of *chronic* disease
  chronic renal disease
  haemoglobinopathy
  bone-marrow failure (e.g. aplastic anaemia or leukaemia).

- Further investigations:
  blood film
  reticulocyte count
  electrophoresis
  serum ferritin (the most useful test for iron deficiency)
  serum vitamin B_{12}
  serum and red cell folate
  renal function tests
  serum bilirubin.

Anaemia with an elevated MCV

This may be due to:
  megaloblastic anaemia, vitamin B_{12} deficiency or folate deficiency
  non-megaloblastic causes (e.g. liver disease, thyroid disease, alcohol, reticulocytosis, myelodysplasia).

- Further investigations:
  blood film
  serum vitamin B_{12}
  serum and red cell folate
  liver function tests
  thyroid function tests.

- Iron deficiency is the commonest cause of anaemia in the UK.

- Chronic illness may be the most common cause of anaemia in the elderly.

- Slow-release iron preparations should not be used to treat anaemia.

- Failure of anaemia to respond to treatment may be due to lack of compliance.

HAEMOLYTIC ANAEMIA

- Haemolysis in the presence of anaemia can be confirmed by the presence of large numbers of reticulocytes on the blood film, and a raised serum bilirubin level.

- The commonest cause of haemolytic anaemia is acute blood loss (usually with normal serum bilirubin level) and liver disease, including biliary obstruction (usually with a raised serum bilirubin level).

SERUM FERRITIN

- This is an iron–protein complex which plays a part in absorption, transport and storage.
- Serum iron and total iron-binding capacity have been largely superseded by serum ferritin.
- Normal range (μg/1):
  adult male, 30–300
  pre-menopausal female, 7–280
  post-menopausal female, 14–230
  children aged 6 months to 15 years, 7–150.
- Serum ferritin is influenced by diet and recent oral therapy.

Abnormal test results

- Low serum ferritin indicates iron deficiency.
- Lowered serum ferritin, lowered folate and low vitamin B_{12} suggest malabsorption.
- Normal or raised serum ferritin suggests
  liver disease
  malignancy
  chronic inflammation (e.g. rheumatoid arthritis (RA)) (yet the iron and total iron-binding capacity may be reduced).
- Raised serum ferritin may be indicative of haemochromatosis, an inborn error of iron metabolism, which may present with vague symptoms, e.g. weakness, lethargy, loss of libido, impotence or weight loss. Organ damage is likely if undetected, e.g. liver damage (cirrhosis/hepatocellular cancer), pancreas (diabetes), arthropathy (chondrocalcinosis), abnormal skin pigmentation, cardiomyopathy and gonadal hypertrophy can all occur.

NB The lower limit of the normal ferritin range is raised in chronic disease (e.g. RA with ferritin of 40 is probably iron deficient.)

SERUM IRON

- Normal range (µg%) is 80–150.
- Ideally, blood should be taken in a fasting state and not while the patient is taking oral iron.
- This is a cheaper investigation than serum ferritin, but gives a less accurate indication of body iron stores.

Abnormal test results

- Lowered serum iron and lowered total iron-binding capacity (TIBC) with normal or raised ferritin suggest anaemia of chronic disease.
- Increased serum iron is seen in:
    iron overload
    contraceptive pill users
    liver disease
    anaemias (e.g. haemolysis)
    haemochromatosis (raised iron, raised serum ferritin, reduced TIBC).

IRON DEFICIENCY ANAEMIA

- This is characterised by low ferritin, low serum iron, raised TIBC, low MCV and low MCHC.
- Blood film may show hypochromasia, anisocytosis, poikilocytosis and pencil cells.
- MCV falls in parallel with Hb and is often lower than in thalassaemia. RBC may be normal.
- Iron deficiency anaemia is caused by:
    blood loss from the gastrointestinal tract
    menorrhagia
    pregnancy
    malabsorption or dietary insufficiency.

NORMOCHROMIC NORMOCYTIC ANAEMIA

- This is characterised by low Hb, normal MCV, normal MCH and normal MCHC.

- It may be caused by:
    chronic disorders (e.g. renal failure, RA)
    pregnancy
    recent blood loss
    haemolysis.

HAEMOLYSIS

- Haemolysis may be congenital:
    sickle-cell disease
    thalassaemia
    congenital spherocytosis
    glucose-6-phosphate dehydrogenase deficiency causing haemolysis with certain drugs (e.g. sulphonamides, nitrofurantoin and quinine).

- Alternatively, it may be acquired:
    infections (e.g. mononucleosis, mycoplasma)
    systemic lupus erythematosus (SLE)
    drugs (e.g. penicillins, cephalosporin, quinine, methyldopa, hydralazine, antimalarials or sulphonamide antibiotics)
    malignancy
    endocrine deficiency
    aplasia
    systemic disease (e.g. liver disease, uraemia).

MACROCYTIC ANAEMIA

- This is characterised by lowered Hb and MCV > 99.

- As well as macrocytes in the blood film, additional features include hypersegmentation of the neutrophils and occasionally leucopenia and thrombocytopenia.

- Macrocytic anaemia is often due to vitamin B_{12} or folate deficiency causing megaloblastic changes in the bone marrow. Vitamin B_{12} deficiency may be dietary (e.g. in Hindu vegetarians, vegans) in origin or due to pernicious anaemia. Folate deficiency may be due to malabsorption or antifolate drugs (e.g. anticonvulsants, trimethoprim or triamterene).

- Macrocytic anaemia may also be due to non-megaloblastic causes:
    alcohol
    liver disease
    myxoedema
    aplastic anaemia
    myeloma.

SERUM FOLATE

- This is usually measured in conjunction with red cell folate.
- Normal range (μg/1) is 2–14 (5–40 nmol/1).
- Red cell folate is a better guide to tissue stores, whilst serum folate indicates the immediate level.

RED CELL FOLATE

- This is usually measured in conjunction with serum folate.
- Normal range (μg/1) is 130–620 (400–1600 nmol/1).
- Red cell folate may be low in vitamin B_{12} deficiency states.

VITAMIN B_{12}

- Normal range (ng/1) is 170–700.
- Low WCC can cause a low B_{12}.
- In pernicious anaemia (PA) levels are often <50.
- 10–15% of people with PA have normal vitamin B_{12} levels.

SERUM INTRINSIC FACTOR ANTIBODY ASSAY

- Normal range (IU/ml) is <2.5.

Abnormal test results

- Lowered serum intrinsic factor antibody assay (<2) suggests a negative result.
- A borderline result (2.5) suggests that a repeat test should be performed.
- Raised serum intrinsic factor antibody assay (>2.5) suggests pernicious anaemia.

RETICULOCYTE COUNT

- If anaemia is present, the reticulocyte count gives an indication of the marrow response.
- Normal range (%) is 0.2–2.
- Peaks occur 3–5 days after the start of treatment with folic acid or vitamin B_{12} and 7 days after treatment with iron.

Abnormal test results

- A raised reticulocyte count suggests:
    haemolysis following haemorrhage
    a response to treatment with haematinics.

PLASMA VISCOSITY

- Measures the flow rate of plasma compared with water.
- Normal range (mPa) is 1.25–1.72.
- Advantages of the plasma viscosity test over erythrocyte sedimentation rate (ESR):
    it is independent of age, sex and Hb level
    plasma can be kept at room temperature for 48 hours without affecting the result (unlike ESR, which must be read within 4 hours)
    steroids *do not* affect the result
    high sensitivity
    few false-negative results
    the test is easily automated
    it is cheap.

Test results

- Reduced plasma viscosity (<1.5) occurs in low plasma proteins.
- Normal range is 1.5–1.72 (up to 1.8 in the third trimester of pregnancy).
- Raised plasma viscosity (1.72–3.0) occurs in acute or chronic disease.
- Raised plasma viscosity (>3.0) strongly suggests myeloma or macroglobulinaemia (levels usually greatly exceed this value).

ERYTHROCYTE SEDIMENTATION RATE (ESR)

- This measurement varies widely in different physiological and pathological conditions.
- The ESR is influenced by age, sex and anaemia and must be measured within 2 hours of venepuncture.
- The 'normal' range varies depending on the technique (e.g. Westergren, Wintrobe or Seditainer).
- The approximate normal range (using the Westergren method) for males is equal to the age in years divided by 2, and for females is equal to the age in years +10 divided by 2.
- The specimen should remain in a vertical position and must be transported to the laboratory immediately.
- If the specimen is refrigerated, it should be allowed to warm to room temperature before testing.

Abnormal test results

- Raised ESR can be found in:
  disease (any acute inflammatory response) e.g. temporal arteritis, though note that the ESR can be normal in temporal arteritis
  pregnancy
  oral contraceptive pill users
  anaemia (falsely evelated result)
  obsesity can cause a moderately raised ESR.

NB Very high (>100) ESR is found in autoimmune disease, malignancy, acute post-trauma and serious infection. A false high ESR can occur if the ambient temperature is unusually high, if the Westergren tube is not held vertically, or if dextran is present in the blood sample.

- Low ESR is found in:
    heart failure
    PRV
    sickle-cell anaemia
    treatment with steroids.

NB A false low ESR can occur if the ambient temperature is unusually low, if the Westergren tube contains air bubbles, or if the tube is dirty.

C-REACTIVE PROTEIN (CRP)

- C-reactive protein is an acute phase protein, so it is elevated in infection (more so with bacterial infection, less elevated with viral infection) and inflammation but not elevated with many malignancies.

- Normal range (mg/1) is <4.

- It changes more rapidly than ESR.

- Levels are increased up to several hundred times following an acute infective or non-infective inflammatory response.

- Elevation may occur in lipaemic sera.

- CRP is sometimes used to monitor the response to second-line drugs in the treatment of RA. Maintaining CRP within the normal range leads to less joint erosion.

- CRP levels are often normal in malignancy.

SERUM HAPTOGLOBIN

- This is a serum protein which combines with Hb.

- Normal range (g/1) is 0.3–2.0.

- It is measured principally in patients in whom acute haemolysis is suspected, when levels may fall below 0.1.

- An increase in haptoglobin occurs in many systemic diseases and inflammatory conditions.

SERUM FIBRINOGEN

- Normal range (g/l) is 1.5–4.0.
- It is measured principally when disseminated intravascular coagulation (DIC) is suspected.
- It is a major risk factor for coronary heart disease (CHD).
- A sodium citrate blood bottle is used.

INFECTIOUS MONONUCLEOSIS

- Infection with the Epstein–Barr virus (EBV) (human herpes type 4 virus) has been implicated in a wide spectrum of clinical diseases, ranging from glandular fever to lymphoma.
- Diagnosis of glandular fever is by the following:
    the *Monospot test* – a rapid, simple slide test for the detection of heterophil antibodies. It is less specific and less sensitive than the Paul Bunnel test, giving negative results for 10–20% of adults with proven infectious mononucleosis and up to 50% of children
    the *Paul Bunnel test* is positive in 80% of patients in the first week of illness and in about 60% of cases by the end of the second week. It may remain negative in 10% of cases, particularly in adolescents and young adults. If the test is negative at the first consultation but the diagnosis of glandular fever is most likely, then the test may be repeated after 7–10 days. The antibody titre is highest during the second and third weeks of the illness, and declines thereafter. The length of time for which the test remains positive thereafter depends on the type of test used, and it may remain positive for up to 1 year. The size and duration of antibody response bears no relationship to the severity of the illness
    the *IgM antibody test* – the Epstein–Han virus IgM antibody appears early in glandular fever, and disappears after 3 months. In young children, IgM may be positive when

the Paul Bunnel test is negative. It is usually only necessary to request antibodies when the illness is very severe.

- Atypical lymphocytes >10% are commonly but not always seen in glandular fever.

- Other viral infections that may cause a lymphocytosis, but which give a negative Paul Bunnel test, include:
    viral hepatitis
    rubella
    toxoplasmosis
    cytomegalovirus (CMV) infection
    HIV infection.

- Liver function tests will often be abnormal in patients with glandular fever, transaminases and bilirubin levels reaching 2–3 times normal in over 80% of patients with glandular fever.

White cell indices

WHITE BLOOD CELL COUNT (WBC)

- Normal range ($\times 10^9/1$) is 4–11.

- The white cell count is similar in males and females, and remains very constant throughout life in 50% of the population.

- More important than the total white cell count is the *differential white cell count*. White cell counts of $>11 \times 10^9/1$ should have a differential white cell count performed.

- The white cell count rarely exceeds $50 \times 10^9/1$ except in leukaemia.

- The total WBC or any individual element may be lowered by steroids.

NB Individuals of Afro-Caribbean origin have a lower normal range.

DIFFERENTIAL WBC

- Normal range ($\times 10^9/1$):
  neutrophils, 2.5–7.5 (60–70%)
  lymphocytes, 1.5–4.0 (25–30%)
  monocytes, 0.2–0.8 (5–10%)
  eosinophils, 0.04–0.44 (1–4%)
  basophils, up to 0.1 (up to 1%).

- Individuals of Afro-Caribbean origin have lower neutrophil counts than those of other races.

NB Young children normally have a reverse differential count, i.e. more lymphocytes than neutrophils.

Abnormal test results

- Cigarette smokers often have high (but normal) white cell counts proportional to the number of cigarettes smoked, presumed to be due to inflammatory lung disease.

- Raised WBC (leucocytosis) is commonly found in:
  bacterial infection
  pregnancy (third trimester)
  post-trauma (e.g. burns, surgery)
  post-haemorrhage
  malignancy
  drugs (e.g. steroids, digoxin, lithium, beta-agonists)
  myeloproliferative disorders
  myocardial infarction (MI)
  renal failure
  gout
  diabetes mellitus.

- A lowered white cell count necessitates a differential white cell count.

- The white cell count may be lowered in:
  viral infections
  bacterial infection (e.g. overwhelming septicaemia, brucellosis, typhoid, miliary tuberculosis)
  drugs (e.g. thiouracil, mianserin, meprobamate and phenylbutazone)

folate or vitamin B_{12} deficiency

autoimmune neutropenia, SLE, Felty's syndrome, post-coronary artery bypass-graft (CABG) and haemodialysis

agranulocytosis (severe leucopenia in an ill patient).

- Agranulocytosis can be caused by:

  drugs that give rise to pancytopenia (e.g. antimitotic drugs and antirheumatic drugs such as gold, as well as carbimazole)

  some malignancies (e.g. leukaemia, non-Hodgkin's lymphoma) may present with low WBC.

- Neutropenia (neutrophils $<1 \times 10^9/1$) may be due to:

  infections (e.g. bacterial/viral tuberculosis (TB), typhoid, brucellosis, rickettsia and malaria)

  drugs (e.g. cytotoxic therapy, some antirheumatic agents, mianserin, carbimazole)

  thyroid disease

  cirrhosis

  hypopituitarism

  aplastic anaemia

  bone-marrow infiltration

  RA

  SLE.

- Patients with severe neutropenia (<1.0) should be referred for investigation.

NB Neutropenia is sometimes found without any cause in Black populations and in some women.

- Eosinophils $>6\%$ (eosinophilia) suggests:

  allergic reactions (e.g. to drugs, parasites)

  polyarteritis

  reticulocytosis

  sarcoidosis

  myeloproliferative disorders

  leukaemia

  erythema multiforme

  irradiation

  congenital causes

  dermatitis herpetiformis

pemphigus
scarlet fever
acute rheumatic fever
rheumatoid arthritis
smoking.

- A very high eosinophil count is seen in some carcinomas, hydatid disease and eosinophilic leukaemia.

- A lowered eosinophil count occurs with corticosteroids and occurs during the early phase of acute insults and shock and trauma surgery.

- A lymphocyte count of >45% (lymphocytosis) is found in some infections (e.g. infectious mononucleosis, infectious hepatitis, cytomegalovirus, toxoplasmosis, TB, brucellosis, syphilis, poisoning with lead, carbon disulfide tetrachloroethane, leukaemia (CLL)) and with some drugs (e.g. aspirin, griseofulvin, haloperidol and phenytoin).

- A reduced lymphocyte count occurs in:
   some infections
   Hodgkin's disease
   TB
   post-irradiation
   systemic lupus
   renal failure
   carcinomatosis
   drugs (e.g. steroids, lithium and methysergide).

- Raised WBC and raised basophils are found in:
   hypothyroidism
   ulcerative colitis.

- Basophilia as part of a generalised leucocytosis can be a manifestation of myeloproliferative disorders (e.g. myelofibrosis, polycythaemia and chronic myeloid leukaemia).

- A raised monocyte count (monocytosis) occurs in:
   infectious mononucleosis
   Hodgkin's disease
   TB
   subacute bacterial endocarditis (SBE)

acute and chronic leukaemia
lymphoma
solid tumours
recovery after agranulocytosis.

- A lowered monocyte count may be found in:
  chronic infection
  treatment with glucocorticoids
  infections producing endotoxins.

Morphological descriptions of neutrophils

- *Shift to the left*: the presence of immature granulocytes. It occurs as a reaction to pyogenic bacterial infection or after burns or haemorrhage.

- *Shift to the right (hypersegmented neutrophils):* the appearance of neutrophils with >5 nuclear lobes. Characteristic of vitamin B_{12} or folate deficiency when accompanied by macrocytosis or renal failure, or as a congenital anomaly in the absence of macrocytosis.

- *Toxic granulation*: seen in infections and other toxic states, and is of no special significance.

- *Leucoerythroblastic anaemia*: occurs in severe infections, myeloproliferative disorders and in cases where infiltration of the bone marrow has occurred. A bone-marrow biopsy is mandatory.

Large unstained cells (LUC)

- This new parameter is included in the automated differential WBC by some laboratories.

- Normal range (%):
  adults, 0–6
  children, 0–10.

- If LUC is >6%, the laboratory will perform a manual differential count.

PANCYTOPENIA

- All elements of cellular elements are reduced (red cells, white cells and platelets).

- It is due to bone-marrow failure or premature destruction of the cells, and may be caused by:
    malignant disease in the marrow
    autoimmune disease (e.g. RA, SLE)
    increased splenic activity or destruction (e.g. portal hypertension); aplastic anaemia, which can be due to drugs (e.g. antithyroids, antidepressants, anticoagulants, antibiotics, antihistamines, tranquillisers and thiazide diuretics)
    PA
    myelodysplastic syndrome (*see* below)
    acute leukaemia.

MYELODYSPLASTIC SYNDROME (MDS)

- This group of disorders is characterised by peripheral blood cytopenias and morphological abnormalities of the blood and marrow. It probably progresses to leukaemia.

- Five categories exist.

- Full blood count and film usually suggest MDS, showing cytopenia and dysplastic morphology. Macrocytosis and abnormal neutrophils are common. A marrow aspiration is required to confirm the diagnosis.

- It is most common in individuals over 50 years of age, unless there has been previous exposure to radio- or chemotherapy.

- Consider MDS in the elderly with refractory anaemia, bruising and occasionally recurrent infections, especially if cytopenia is present.

- Red cells, platelets and granulocytes may all be affected, or any combination or only one cell type may be involved (e.g. patients may present with a macrocytosis without the anaemia). In the absence of vitamin B_{12} or folate deficiency or hypothyroidism, pre-leukaemia may be suspected.

- A persistent monocytosis in the absence of TB or SBE may be a precursor of pre-leukaemia.

- Bone-marrow examination is required to make the diagnosis.

- Treatment is by transfusion; treat any infection.

- The expected survival period is 2 years, but it can range from 2–3 months to 10 years.

Special types of MDS

- *Sideroblastic anaemia*: white cells and platelets are normal; responds to pyridoxine and folate.

- *Chronic myelomonocytic leukaemia*: monocytosis and splenomegaly.

CHRONIC LYMPHATIC LEUKAEMIA (CLL)

- Chronic lymphatic leukaemia is fairly common, particularly in the elderly.

- Presentation may be insidious, with an unexplained lympho-cytosis.

- A lymphocyte count of $>15 \times 10^9/1$ requires referral to a haema-tologist for further investigation.

- In CLL there is often a normochromic normocytic anaemia.

- WCC may range from $50–200 \times 10^9/l$.

- Decreased platelets.

- There are five stages of CLL:
    - 0, lymphocytosis, normal marrow function except for increased lymphocytes
    - 1, lymphadenopathy in addition to the above
    - 2, splenomegaly plus lymphadenopathy or hepatomegaly
    - 3–4, either Hb <10 or platelets <100, indicating impaired bone-marrow function.

- The prognosis is good for patients in stages 0–2 of the disease and poor for patients in stages 3 and 4 (about 2–3 years).

DRUGS CAUSING BLOOD DYSCRASIAS

- Idiosyncratic blood dyscrasias include neutropenia, thrombocytopenia and aplastic anaemia caused by a direct toxic effect on cell production by the drug or its metabolites.

- The incidence of blood dyscrasias increases with age of the patient, dose of the drug and duration of use of the drug. Renal or hepatic impairment and the concomitant use of other cytotoxic drugs will also increase the likelihood of reactions.

Neutropenia	Thrombocytopenia	Aplastic anaemia
Captopril	Heparin	NSAIDs
Phenothiazines	Anticonvulsants	Anticonvulsants
Carbimazole	Gold	Gold
Sulphonamides	Sulphonamides	Sulphonamides
Clozapine	Rifampicin	Chloramphenicol
Mianserin	Quinine/quinidine	Penicillamine
Propylthiouracil		Phenothiazines

- Haemolytic anaemias may also occur when using penicillins, methyldopa, hydralazine, anti-malarials or sulphonamide antibiotics.

Platelets

- Normal range ($\times 10^9/1$) is 150–400.

Abnormal test results

- Low platelet counts are found in:
    bone-marrow hypoplasia/aplasia
    bone-marrow infiltration
    vitamin B_{12}/folate deficiency
    immune thrombocytopenia, including drugs (e.g. thiazides, gold, quinidine, sulphonamides)
    infections

hypersplenism

DIC

ITP

severe infections

following massive haemorrhage

liver disease/alcohol

uraemia

patients who have received many blood transfusions

idiopathy.

- Increased platelet counts are found in:

  trauma

  infection and inflammation (e.g. chronic inflammatory bowel disease)

  malignancy and myeloproliferative disorders (e.g. myelofibrosis, essential thrombocythaemia, chronic leukaemia)

  rebound thrombocytosis, which occurs after haemorrhage, haemolysis and post-splenectomy

  post-exercise.

- Giant platelets may be seen in a blood film, and may occur following any acute illness or haemorrhage. They may also precede some forms of leukaemia. In an otherwise healthy person with this finding, the test should be repeated in 4–6 weeks.

Blood coagulation tests

- A family and drug history is essential, and the following clotting and bleeding time tests may be of help.

- Acquired clotting defects are more common than congenital ones.

- In patients who present with bruising or frank bleeding, clotting disorders should be considered.

- Purpura, which is characterised by flat, sharp-edged, dark red lesions which do not blanch on pressure, may be caused by thrombocytopenia or increased vascular fragility, as in senile purpura or patients on long-term steroid therapy, or with Cushing's disease.

- About 70% of patients who present with bruising will have no haematological abnormality.
- Anticoagulation therapy is the commonest cause of acquired bleeding disorders. Warfarin therapy affects factors II, VII, IX and X.
- Liver disease can also cause abnormal bleeding via a number of mechanisms.
- Of the inherited disorders associated with abnormal bleeding, haemophilia (which includes haemophilia A, due to factor VIII deficiency, and haemophilia B, due to factor IX deficiency, and also known as Christmas disease) is the commonest.
- Infiltrative disease of the bone marrow, seen in aplastic anaemia, leukaemia and malignant disease, can produce thrombocytopenia, which may also be caused by some drugs, such as thiazide diuretics, quinine, quinidine, methyldopa, digoxin, and some infections (e.g. rubella, glandular fever and mumps).
- Acute idiopathic thrombocytopenic purpura is most commonly seen 2–3 weeks after an upper respiratory infection. In children, especially boys, Henoch–Schonlein purpura may present with a rash, most commonly distributed on the extensor surfaces and buttocks, accompanied by fever, myalgia, joint pains, abdominal pain and glomerulonephritis.
- Acute idiopathic thrombocytopenic purpura will present 5–10 times in the average GP's career.
- Vascular causes of purpura include senile purpura, cough purpura in children with whooping cough, and rare connective tissue disorders.

PLASMA FIBRINOGEN

- Normal range (g/1) is 1.5–4.0 (0.2–0.4%).

Abnormal test results

- Decreased levels are found in:
  liver disease
  DIC.
- Increased levels are found:
  following tissue damage or infection
  in pregnancy
  in nephrotic syndrome
  in collagen disease.

- Patients with high plasma fibrinogen levels (>3.5 g/l) as well as high serum cholesterol (>6.2 mmol/l) and a systolic blood pressure of >140 mmHg have a 12-fold higher incidence of heart attack than do those with a fibrinogen level of <2.9 g/l. Reducing weight and cholesterol, as well as stopping smoking, lowers fibrinogen – as do clofibrate and bezafibrate.

FIBRIN DEGRADATION PRODUCTS (FDP)

- Normal range (mg/1) is <10.

Abnormal test results

- Raised levels are found in:
  increased fibrinolysis such as post-MI, deep vein thrombosis
      (DVT), pulmonary embolism (PE) and DIC
  liver or renal failure (secondary to DIC).

ACTIVATED PARTIAL THROMBOPLASTIN TIME

- Also known as kaolin cephalin clotting time (KCCT).

- Normal range is 26–39 seconds: laboratory reference >40±7 is abnormal and always requires investigation.

- A measurement of the intrinsic side of the clotting factor cascade.

- This is the most suitable test for monitoring IV heparin, but not subcutaneously.

- APTT, normal range 1.5–2.5 for someone on heparin therapy.

Abnormal test results

- Prolonged KCCT occurs in the following:
  heparin therapy
  clotting factor deficiency syndromes (usually factors VIII and IX, and occasionally factors XI and XII, e.g. Von Willebrand's disease)
  presence of clotting inhibiting factors, such as may be present in the para-proteinaemias or lupus
  liver disease
  after massive transfusions.

PROTHROMBIN TIME

- This is one of the tests used to monitor oral anticoagulants.
- Normal range (sec) is control ±4 (usually 13–15).
- It tests the extrinsic clotting system (factors II, VII and X).
- The result is inversely proportional to the prothrombin content of the blood tested.

INTERNATIONAL NORMALISED RATIO (INR)

See section below on warfarin in practice.

- The INR is the ratio of the patient's prothrombin time (the time taken for plasma to form a fibrin clot when mixed with tissue thromboplastin) and the control prothrombin time raised to the power of the International Sensitivity Index.
- An INR of 1 represents the clotting time of an individual with normal clotting. An INR of 2 indicates that the sample of blood takes twice as long to clot.

Thrombo test

- This is used in some centres to measure warfarin therapy.
- Normal range (%) is 7–17.

Warfarin in practice

Warfarin antagonises vitamin K, leading to depletion of several clotting factors and the inhibition of thrombin formation. The full anticoagulant effect takes 24 to 48 hours to develop, so heparin must be given concurrently if an immediate effect is required. Warfarin is commonly used in the prevention and treatment of venous thrombo-embolism, the prevention of embolism from a mechanical heart valve prosthesis, or in the presence of atrial fibrillation complicating rheumatic valvular disease and, increasingly, in patients with non-rheumatic atrial fibrillation.

CONTROL

The warfarin dosage is adjusted according to the INR (*see* p. 29), which should be measured before warfarin is started. The recommended starting dose in acute situations is 10 mg daily for 2 days, and less for those with heart failure, the very elderly and patients with impaired liver function. Initially, the INR should be measured on alternate days, with progressive lengthening of the interval as control is established. *The interval between tests should never exceed 8 weeks.* In non-urgent situations (e.g. the presence of non-rheumatic atrial fibrillation), a more gradual introduction of warfarin at a dose of 4 mg daily may be preferable and reduces the required frequency of INR tests. The maintenance dose of warfarin is best taken at the same time each day.

The commonest cause of unexpected test results is non-compliance with the recommended warfarin dosage.

For the prophylaxis of DVT, including surgery on high-risk patients, a target range of 2.0–2.5 is advised.

In the treatment of DVT or PE the target INR is 2–3, and in the presence of a mechanical heart valve prosthesis the INR target range is 3.0–4.5.

In the case of some bileaflet valve prostheses, particularly in the aortic position, some authorities recommend a target INR in the lower part of this range, i.e. 2–3, but not below.

Studies among patients with non-rheumatic atrial fibrillation suggest that a target INR of 2.0 may be sufficient to provide protection against stroke. In the presence of previous cerebral ischaemia, a target ratio of 2.0 to 3.9 has been advised.

IMPORTANT DRUG INTERACTIONS

A large number of drugs can either potentiate or antagonise the anticoagulant effect of warfarin by interfering with absorption or metabolism either of the drug or of vitamin K.

Drugs that are likely to potentiate the anticoagulant effect of warfarin

These include alcohol, aspirin, non-steroidal anti-inflammatory drugs (NSAIDs), steroids, amiodarone, propafenone, some antibiotics (ciprofloxacin, co-trimoxazole, sulphonamides, erythromycin, aminoglycosides, metronidazole and possibly ampicillin), fibrates, simvastatin, thyroxine, dextropropoxyphene, dipyridamole, miconazole, ketoconazole, allopurinol, cimetidine, danazol and some antidepressants.

Drugs that are likely to antagonise the anticoagulant effect of warfarin

These include oral contraceptives, some anti-epileptics (carbamazepine and primidone, phenytoin), griseofulvin and rifampicin.

In addition, *major dietary changes can influence the anticoagulant effect of warfarin*, such as a substantial increase in alcohol (which enhances the effect) or in vegetable consumption (which antagonises it). When in doubt (e.g. during a prolonged course of treatment involving antibiotics or a NSAID), or if there is a substantial change in the patient's health (particularly an increase in heart failure or a febrile illness), it is important to increase the frequency of INR checks.

DENTISTRY

Dental surgery may be undertaken in most patients with little risk of haemorrhage if the INR is ≤ 2.0. More major surgery requires that the relative risks of stopping warfarin or continuing with anti-coagulants throughout the operative period be assessed on an individual patient basis by the specialist team concerned.

PREGNANCY

Warfarin crosses the placenta and between weeks 6 and 9 it is teratogenic (nasal hypoplasia – stippled epiphyses). It may also cause fetal haemorrhage, particularly in the third trimester. None the less, maintenance of warfarin therapy may represent the safest option in some circumstances (e.g. pregnant women with diseased or prosthetic heart valves).

Heparin may be given subcutaneously and does not cross the placenta. It may cause thrombocytopenia and osteoporosis if given for more than 6 months.

DURATION OF TREATMENT WITH WARFARIN

Up to 12 months

- Prophylaxis of DVT, including high-risk surgery.
- Treatment of an established venous thrombosis.
- Treatment of an established pulmonary embolus.
- MI, anterior myocardial infarct (usually a minimum of 3 months of treatment with warfarin).
- Xenograft heart valve replacement.
- CABG.

Lifelong treatment with warfarin

- Recurrent venous thrombo-embolism.
- Embolic complications of rheumatic heart disease and atrial fibrillation.
- Cardiac prosthetic valve replacement and arterial grafts.

Thrombophilia

- This is an inherited or acquired tendency towards abnormal clotting.

- It is two to three times more common than bleeding disorders.

- Recent adverse publicity regarding the increased risk of thrombosis in women taking certain newer, third-generation oral contraceptive pills should result in the referral of all such women with a positive family history of thrombosis.

- Consider thrombophilia in people under 40 years of age with recurrent thrombo-embolic disease or a primary thrombo-embolic event with a strong family history.

- Check antithrombin III, protein C and protein S, lupus anticoagulant and anticardiolipin antibodies, as well as disorders of fibrinolysis.

- A positive family history may be present, and should lead to screening of other at-risk relatives.

- Other predisposing factors for thrombosis coexist in 50% of cases.

- Refer the patient to a haematologist.

NB Thrombophilic patients who suffer thrombotic episodes will need long-term prophylaxis with warfarin.

MANAGEMENT OF PATIENTS WITH THROMBOPHILIA

Patients who have a tendency to thrombosis do so because they have a disorder of the blood (e.g. a coagulation defect or a cellular abnormality such as polycythaemia) or a defect of the vessel wall. Where enhanced coagulation is the primary cause, the disorder is referred to as thrombophilia.

In patients with thrombophilia, the mechanisms that normally inhibit thrombosis are impaired, resulting, for example, in thrombosis at an early age or recurrent thrombosis. The risk of thrombosis is increased by obesity, immobility, trauma, pregnancy and malignancy. Thrombophilia may be inherited or acquired.

INHERITED THROMBOPHILIA

Inherited resistance to activated protein C2 and inherited deficiencies of antithrombin III, protein C and protein S predispose to thrombosis. Inherited resistance to activated protein C occurs in up to 7% of the population and produces a variant factor V (factor V Leiden) which, when detected in women, can indicate a predisposition to thrombosis during pregnancy and while taking the oral contraceptive pill.

ACQUIRED THROMBOPHILIA

The most frequent cause of acquired thrombophilia is the antiphospholipid syndrome, which is caused by the presence of lupus anticoagulant and/or anticardiolipin antibody predisposing to venous and arterial thrombosis.

WHO SHOULD BE INVESTIGATED?

The following observations should alert the physician to the possibility of thrombophilia:

- venous thrombo-embolism in a patient aged under 40 years
- recurrent venous thrombosis or thrombophlebitis
- venous thrombosis in an unusual site (e.g. mesenteric or cerebral vein)
- skin necrosis, especially in a patient taking warfarin
- arterial thrombosis in a patient aged under 30 years
- a family history of venous thrombo-embolism
- recurrent fetal loss
- unexplained neonatal thrombosis.

INVESTIGATIONS

These should include the following:

- full blood count, including platelet count
- prothrombin time
- activated partial thromboplastin time
- thrombin time
- reptilase time
- fibrinogen concentration.

These tests will detect polycythaemia, thrombocytosis and dysfibrinogenaemia and suggest the presence of the lupus anticoagulant. If thrombophilia is still suspected, detailed further investigations are required.

Haemoglobinopathies

Because many inherited haemoglobin and red-cell enzyme disorders confer partial protection against malaria, haemoglobinopathies are more common in ethnic groups that originate from endemic malaria zones. In the UK, patients of Afro-Caribbean, Asian and Mediterranean origin are more likely to carry the genetic disorders.

SICKLE-CELL DISEASE (SCD)

- Haemolysis may lead to anaemia and increased folic acid requirements.
- It mainly affects people of African, Afro-Caribbean, Middle Eastern and Mediterranean descent.
- About 5000 people are affected in the UK, with many more having the sickle-cell trait.
- The clinical syndromes have variable penetration, and some individuals are more affected than others.

- Infants born with SCD are at high risk of death due to over-whelming pneumococcal infection. Symptoms are rarely present during the first 6 months of life, due to the presence of fetal Hb, but often appear during the first 2 years of life, as fetal Hb levels decrease. The affected infant suffers from recurrent respiratory infections, failure to thrive and anaemia. Chronic haemolysis leads to anaemia (Hb is often around 8 g/dl, with 10–30% reticulocytes). Pulmonary complications, stroke and meningitis are common causes of death.

- The diagnosis is made by electrophoresis.

- Other children and adults often present with pain 'crises', such as repeated episodes of asymmetrical joint or bone pain, sometimes associated with abdominal or chest pain.

THALASSAEMIA

- This is the most common haemoglobinopathy, affecting 4% of the world's population and 5% of the population of England and Wales.

- It is the most common inherited disease in the UK among immigrants from the Mediterranean, East Africa, Asia (including South-East Asia and Vietnam) and the Caribbean.

- Two forms exist, depending on which globin chain is affected (alpha or beta). Beta-thalassaemia can be divided into major (found in those who have the disease) and minor (found in those who carry the disease).

- Thalassaemia confers protection against *Plasmodium falciparum* (malaria).

Beta-thalassaemia major

- It begins in early childhood.

- Severe anaemia leads to frequent blood transfusions.

- Bony deformities appear due to expansion of the bone-marrow cavities.

- Splenomegaly occurs.

- Tissue hypoxia, iatrogenic iron overload resulting in liver damage, cardiac failure and endocrine failure usually result in death before the age of 30 years.

- Patients should receive regular iron chelation therapy with subcutaneous desferrioxamine.

Thalassaemia minor (the carrier state)

- This is asymptomatic, although it may be suspected when a blood film shows a microcytic hypochromic anaemia with target cells, poikilocytosis and basophil stippling, together with a normal serum ferritin (unlike iron deficiency, where the ferritin would also be lowered).

- The importance of thalassaemia minor is in the prevention of the homozygous thalassaemia major.

- Hb is often 10–15 g/dl, whilst RBC is higher and MCH and MCHC are lower than in comparable cases of iron deficiency anaemia.

Alpha-thalassaemia

- This is distinguished from beta-thalassaemia by electrophoresis.

GLUCOSE-6-PHOSPHATE DEHYDROGENASE DEFICIENCY

This affects ethnic groups similar to those affected by thalassaemia and can lead to severe haemolytic disease. The gene is carried on the X-chromosome, so usually only males are affected. The Mediterranean type may lead to *favism*, namely acute intravascular haemolysis following the ingestion of certain types of bean.

Glucose-6-phosphate dehydrogenase deficiency renders affected individuals susceptible to haemolysis produced by certain oxidant drugs and infections.

Laboratory findings

- Haemoglobinopathies and glucose-6-phosphate dehydrogenase deficiency often show a microcytic anaemia.
- In the thalassaemia trait there is often a low MCV and MCHC and high red cell count.
- Target cells may be seen.
- Electrophoresis is diagnostic.

Effects of drug therapies on blood

- Many second-line drugs that are used in the treatment of RA can have serious adverse effects on bone marrow and liver function tests (LFTs).
- Before starting treatment, a full blood count, ESR, initial profile and LFTs should be monitored as a baseline.
- Full blood count and LFTs are usually assessed monthly for the first 6 months of treatment, and 3-monthly thereafter.

ROUTINE TESTING OF PATIENTS RECEIVING DISEASE MODIFYING ANTIRHEUMATIC DRUGS

Drug	Test
Penicillamine	FBC and urinary protein weekly then monthly
Azathioprine	FBC monthly
Gold	FBC and urinary protein and blood prior to each gold injection
Sulphasalazine	FBC every 2 weeks LFTs before and monthly, then 3-monthly after commencing drug

Methotrexate

FBC monthly, creatinine and LFTs before starting and 3-monthly

Hydroxychloroquine

Full ophthalmic examination every 3–6 months

STOP the above drugs if the following occur:

WBC $< 3.5 \times 10^9/l$

Platelets $< 120 \times 10^9/l$

LFTs $> 3 \times$ normal range

Consult rheumatologist if
    LFTs $> 1.5 \times$ normal range

Urinary protein $> 1g/24$ hours

Microscopic haematuria on
    dipstick testing

Macrocytosis or abrupt fall in
    blood count in patients on
    methotrexate

GOLD, PENICILLAMINE (DISTAMINE, PENDRAMINE) AND AURANOFIN (RIDAURA)

- These may cause eosinophilia (> 0.04–0.44) (1–4%). Stop gold therapy for 1–2 weeks and then resume it at a lower dose.

- A trace of protein or blood can be ignored. If it occurs on more than one consecutive occasion, perform a mid-stream urine test (MSU) and withhold gold therapy until it clears.

- Withhold gold therapy if WBC is $< 3.5 \times 10^9/l$ or neutrophil count is $< 2 \times 10^9/l$ or platelet count is $< 120 \times 10^9/l$.

- A high platelet count ($> 400 \times 10^9/l$) is sometimes a sign of active RA and falls with treatment.

- Sore throat, severe mouth ulcers or a high temperature may indicate serious neutropenia. Drugs should be stopped and an immediate WBC performed.

CYCLOSPORIN (NEORAL AND SANDIMMUN)

- This is an immunosuppressive agent.

- It is used in the treatment of severe psoriasis and eczema.

- Check blood pressure and serum creatinine levels every 2 weeks during the initial 3 months, and then monthly if the patient is stable.

- If creatinine increases to >30% above the patient's baseline, then reduce the dose.

- The baseline glomerular filtration rate (GFR) should be measured and the measurement repeated within 2 months of the start of therapy.

- Initial and periodic measurement of bilirubin, liver enzymes, potassium, magnesium, uric acid and urinary protein are all required.

Common haematological terms

ANISOCYTES (RED CELLS OF VARIABLE SIZE)

- Abnormally shaped cells that are sometimes associated with megaloblastic anaemia, partially treated iron deficiency and some conditions in which the anaemia is secondary to systemic disease.

POIKILOCYTOSIS (RED CELLS OF VARIABLE SHAPE)

- Tear-shaped cells suggestive of an erythropoiesis defect that are seen in megaloblastic anaemias and myelofibrosis.

SPHEROCYTES

- Abnormally thick red cells that are associated with:
    hereditary spherocytosis
    haemolytic disorders

severe burns
Clostridium welchii septicaemia.

ELIPTOCYTES

- Pencil-shaped cells that are seen in:
    iron deficiency anaemia
    mild congenital haemolytic anaemia.

TARGET CELLS

- Cells that are associated with:
    iron deficiency
    anaemia
    haemoglobinopathy (including thalassaemia, liver disorders
        and splenectomy).

SPUR CELLS

- Cells that are seen in severe hepatic disease.

BURR CELLS

- Irregularly contracted red cells that are seen in renal disease.

FRAGMENTED RED CELLS

- Cells that are seen:
    in DIC
    post-splenectomy
    in patients with a heart valve prosthesis.

CRENATION

- Curly or wavy-edged red cells – sometimes indicative of renal
  disease. Therefore urea and electrolytes are appropriate as the
  next investigation.
- Crenation occurs:
    in hypothyroidism

as an artefact
in the elderly.

HYPOCHROMASIA

- The condition in which cells take stain less readily/intensely than usual.
- It is a feature of:
  iron deficiency
  thalassaemia
  lead poisoning.

POLYCHROMASIA

- Red cells staining slightly blue, associated with an increased number of reticulocytes.
- It *always implies pathology*, and is found in:
  haemolytic anaemia
  haemorrhage
  response to haematinics
  marrow infiltration
  severe hypoxia.

DIMORPHIC RED CELLS

- These may be a feature of sideroblastic anaemia and may also be seen in patients being treated for anaemia secondary to haematinics deficiency, and in patients post-transfusion.

ANISOCYTOSIS

- Variation in the size of red cells.

ECHINOCYTES

- Multiple spicules on the red-cell surface, usually associated with mild haemolysis.

ACANTHOCYTES

- Irregularly contracted red cells, seen in liver disease.

ROULEAUX

- Stacks of red cells in the blood film reflected by an increase in the ESR.
- They may be present in:
  acute infections
  conditions where abnormal plasma proteins are present (e.g. myeloma).

ETHYLENEDIAMINETETRA-ACETIC ACID (EDTA) CHANGES

- Potassium (K^+) EDTA is the anticoagulant of choice for blood counting and enables some of the elements of the blood, especially the platelets, to remain stable for several days.
- The Hb content of a sample does not vary with time even if haemolysis occurs.
- Some changes occur in the white cells (in particular, neutrophils disintegrate), hence the total WBC will be affected and an apparent neutropenia or lymphocytosis may occur.

HEINZ BODIES

- These may be found in haemolytic states, especially when drug-induced.

PANCYTOPENIA

- This may be due to:
  bone-marrow failure
  premature destruction of cells
  malignant disease
  haematological and non-haematological disease (e.g. RA, SLE, myelodysplasia, PA)
  increased splenic activity or destruction (e.g. portal hypertension)

aplastic anaemia, which can be due to drugs (e.g. antithyroids, antidepressants, antibiotics, antihistamines, tranquillisers, thiazide diuretics).

Blood tests in heart failure

- Always do:
  urinalysis
  full blood count
  urea creatinine and electrolytes
  serum glucose.
- Consider:
  LFTs
  CRP
  TSH
  uric acid
  troponin T (to exclude acute myocardial infarction).

2
MICROBIOLOGY

Gastrointestinal organisms

- Examination for ova, cysts and parasites is usually performed routinely.
- All infectious diarrhoea is notifiable as dysentery or food poisoning to the Consultant in Communicable Disease Control (CCDC) in order to locate and eradicate the source.
- Stool specimens should be sent to the laboratory in a sterile, screw-cap container. More than one specimen may be helpful in the identification of organisms such as *Giardia lamblia*.
- Transport the specimen to the laboratory as soon as possible.
- An appropriate plastic container should be used so that dehydration of the specimen is avoided.
- Stool specimens which are to be examined for mobile trophozites should be kept at room temperature and examined shortly after collection, while the organisms are still active.
- Examination of faeces for ova or cysts can be done on a 'cold' specimen.

FOOD POISONING

- The organisms most commonly found are those of the salmonella group, such as *Salmonella typhimurium* and *S. enteritidis*.
- Food poisoning is also commonly caused by *S. aureus* and *Bacillus cereus*, which produce an exotoxin. Occasionally,

Clostridium perfringens and, rarely, *Cl. botulinum* may be the causative organisms.

- The following should be sent to the laboratory in suspected cases:
    portion of food suspected
    stools as soon as these have been passed.

SALMONELLA

Transmission

- This is mainly from food (raw meat, poultry and eggs); rarely from person to person.

Presentation

- Diarrhoea predominates; abdominal pain, vomiting and fever may occur.

Treatment

- Ill or toxic patients require admission to an infectious diseases hospital.
- Patients usually require supportive treatment only, i.e. fluids.

NB Treatment with certain antibiotics can limit the duration of excretion and may be required in severe cases.

SHIGELLA

- Stool samples should be delivered fresh to the laboratory.

Transmission

- This occurs via flies, fingers, food and faeces.

Presentation

- The same symptoms as are caused by *Salmonella* (diarrhoea predominates).

- Common in young children (<8 years), particularly those attending junior schools and nurseries.
- Occasionally the patient may become unwell or toxic.

Treatment

- If the patient is unwell, symptomatic treatment should be given.
- Exclude infected children from school until the diarrhoea has resolved.
- Septrin is rarely indicated.

GIARDIA LAMBLIA (GIARDIA INTESTINALIS)

- Three stool specimens may be required at 24-hour intervals, as cysts are only excreted intermittently.

Transmission

- This is mainly via contaminated water or faeco-oral spread. The organism may be found in stools, especially if the patient has recently returned from abroad having contracted persistent diarrhoea.
- Spread may be rapid in nurseries and junior schools, where faeco-oral spread predominates.

Presentation

- Fatty, offensive and persistent diarrhoea (malabsorption type).

Treatment

- Flagyl daily for 3 days:
    adult, 2 g
    7–10 years, 1 g
    3–7 years, 600 mg.

CLOSTRIDIUM DIFFICILE

- Can cause acute or persistent diarrhoea after prolonged antibiotic use.

VIBRIO CHOLERAE

- This requires a special culture medium and will not be looked for by laboratories unless there is a history of travel to an endemic area (usually the tropics).

Transmission

- This is via water or food contaminated with sewage, the unclean hands of a person with cholera, or by flies. Person-to-person transmission is rare.

Presentation

- Profuse watery diarrhoea and occasionally vomiting. Dehydration may lead to collapse.

CAMPYLOBACTER JEJUNI

- The most common cause of bacterial diarrhoea.
- Requires 48 hours' incubation.

Transmission

- Unpasteurised milk and stream water are often implicated, but it is quite common for the source to remain unidentified.
- Campylobacter is found in the gut and carcass of chickens and other animals, and can be spread during their preparation.
- Person-to-person transmission is rare.

Presentation

- Abdominal pain (sometimes severe abdominal cramps), diarrhoea and feeling generally unwell for up to 2 weeks. Vomiting is uncommon.

Treatment

- Rarely requires treatment.
- Erythromycin may be used, especially if the patient is immuno-supressed or there are severe abdominal cramps.

HELICOBACTER PYLORI

- This is associated with chronic gastritis and relapsing duodenal ulcers. It cannot be isolated from stool culture, but can be grown from gastric biopsy at endoscopy or its presence deduced from a radioisotope CO_2 breath test. An exhaled breath test with a value of <0.25 suggests that no *Helicobacter pylori* is present, whereas a value of >0.25 suggests that *Helicobacter* is present.
- Can be eradicated with Flagyl, amoxycillin and a proton-pump inhibitor.
- The treatment of proven cases of known peptic ulceration remains controversial.

CRYPTOSPORIDIUM (PARVUM)

- This protozoan is common in animal faeces.
- Sometimes seen in young children who have contact with young animals (e.g. on school trips to a farm or in contaminated mains water supplies).

Transmission

- This is via infected cattle, milk or water (especially swimming pools).

Presentation

- Self-limiting gastroenteritis in normal individuals, or it may even be asymptomatic.
- Life-threatening diarrhoea in immunologically depressed individuals.

Treatment

- No effective treatment is available.
- The infection is usually self-limiting, but in immunocompromised patients (e.g. those with AIDS) it may be life-threatening.

ENTEROPATHOGENIC *E. COLI*

- This is detectable using specific agglutination tests.

VIRAL CAUSES OF GASTROENTERITIS

- These can be identified using an electron microscope, or enzyme-linked immunosorbent assay (ELISA) if available. Rotavirus and small round viruses are the most commonly detected organisms.

ENTEROBIUS VERMICULARIS (PINWORM, THREADWORM OR SEATWORM)

- Diagnosis is best made with a Sellotape slide collecting eggs at the perianal margin.

Treatment

- Piperazine:
    6 years to adult: 1 sachet
    1–5 years: $^2/_3$ sachet
    3 months–1 year: $^1/_3$ sachet.
- Repeat after 14 days.
- The whole family should be treated as well as the affected individual.
- It is important to cut and scrub fingernails and to change underclothing and bed linen.

LISTERIOSIS

Transmission

- This is via contaminated food, especially soft cheese, unpasteurised dairy products, chicken and pre-packed salads.

- The organism can grow at refrigeration temperatures (4°C).

Presentation

- Infection is mainly seen in the very young, the very old, pregnant women and the immunocompromised.

- In healthy people, the illness resembles a mild influenza and the diagnosis is rarely made.

- In pregnant women, it may affect the fetus and can lead to miscarriage, stillbirth or severe illness in the newborn infant.

NB A definitive microbiological diagnosis of listeriosis in pregnancy can only be made from a blood culture. Check with the laboratory to ensure that the correct culture is used. Blood cultures should be sent to the laboratory as soon as possible and not refrigerated.

Procedure

- It is very important that any request form accompanying samples from a patient in whom listeriosis is suspected should state this fact clearly. Clinical samples may not be routinely examined for *Listeria*.

Treatment

- A variety of antibiotics, including ampicillin, erythromycin and tetracycline, are used to treat listeriosis.

INVESTIGATIONS THAT CAN HELP DIAGNOSE TRAVEL-RELATED INFECTIONS

- Blood
  FBC with differential white cell count and thick and thin blood films for malarial parasites
  ESR and CRP
  LFTs
  Viral serology including hepatitis serology.

- Urine
  MSU and request examination for ova, cysts and parasites if schistosomiasis is suspected.

- Faeces
  for ova, cysts and parasites.

Urogenital organisms

NB Swabs must be taken from appropriate sites, e.g. vaginal fornices or endocervical, and appropriately labelled and sent in the correct culture medium.

The high vaginal swab (HVS) is not good at detecting gonococcus but may detect trichomonas, candida and bacterial vaginosis. At room temperature a HVS will keep for 24 hours before culture, but it will be unsuitable for testing for gonococci after 12 hours.

- Many different organisms may be present at the same time.

- Refer to genito-urinary clinic for most appropriate investigations and contact tracing.

- Culture of some organisms is difficult, and a specific culture medium must be used.

- In cases of suspected pelvic inflammatory disease (PID), an endocervical swab should be taken for *Neisseria gonorrhoeae* (only a 40% detection rate) and placed in the correct medium, and a further swab taken for *Chlamydia* in the chlamydia transport medium.

- In men, a cotton-tipped wire swab should be taken from 3–4 cm inside the urethra and sent to the laboratory in a transport medium.

HERPES GENITALIS

- This is a common cause of genital ulceration.

Presentation

- In men, an erythematous red area develops, usually on the prepuce, followed by vesicles.
- In women, the most common sites of vesicles are the labia majora and minora, cervix and perineum.

Diagnosis

- This is confirmed by sending material from the ulcer in virus transport medium for culture, although herpes will survive in Stuart's transport medium.
- Differential diagnosis includes primary chancre of syphilis, secondary infection after scratching scabies lesions and trauma secondary to sexual intercourse.

Treatment

- Analgesics for pain relief.
- Zovirax cream 5% and oral Zovirax 200 mg × 5 od for 5 days.
- In frequently recurrent herpes, prophylaxis with oral Zovirax 200 mg 1–4 times daily.

GONORRHOEA

- About 60% of affected women are asymptomatic.
- Dysuria in a young man with a normal urinary tract is more likely to be due to urethritis than to urinary tract infection (UTI).

Presentation

- In men, there is discomfort in the urethra followed by a creamy, thick, yellow-green, purulent discharge.
- In women, there is a vaginal discharge, dysuria, frequency of micturition, backache or abdominal pain.
- *Trichomonas* also present in 50% of positive cases.

Diagnosis

- In men, a swab of urethral discharge should be sent for staining, microscopic examination and culture.
- In women, swabs from the urethra and cervix should be sent for culture.
- Swabs should be transported in Stuart's medium in a bottle with a screw top, or as charcoal swabs.

Treatment

- Seek advice from a genito-urinary clinic with regard to further treatment and contact tracing.
- A single dose of 2.4 mega-units of procaine penicillin, or 3 g ampicillin or 3 g amoxycillin in a single dose, each with probenecid 2 g orally, should be given.
- For patients who are allergic to pencillin, or in cases where there is a high incidence (>5%) of penicillinase-producing *Neisseria gonorrhoeae*, treat with spectinomycin, 2 g IM, or kanamycin, 2 g IM.
- Single-dose ciprofloxacin may be effective.

TRICHOMONAS VAGINALIS

- This is a microscopic parasite.
- It may be an incidental finding on a cervical smear.
- It may occur in association with other venereal diseases.
- Infection may be asymptomatic.

Presentation

- In men, the urethra or its extensions may be infected and cause reinfection of the partner.
- In women, there is a frothy vaginal discharge with vaginal tenderness, swollen and inflamed vulva, and pain on urination.

Diagnosis

- A diagnosis must be made before any treatment is given.
- Mix discharge from the vagina with warm saline solution and examine under the microscope to detect parasites.
- *Trichomonas vaginalis* can be cultured.

Treatment

- If symptomatic, give Flagyl 200 mg tds × 1 week or a 2 g single dose.

GARDNERELLA VAGINALIS OR BACTERIAL VAGINOSIS (PREVIOUSLY KNOWN AS *HAEMOPHILUS VAGINALIS*)

- Bacterial vaginosis is a change in vaginal flora. It is a vaginal infection caused by a mixed group of organisms including *Gardnerella vaginalis*, *Mycoplasma hominis* and anaerobic organisms.

Presentation

- In women, there is a smelly, greyish, irritant vaginal discharge.
- It may be itchy.
- There is a fishy-smelling odour.

Diagnosis

- The diagnosis of bacterial vaginosis is made when three out of four of the following are present:

a smelly, greyish, irritant vaginal discharge, which may be itchy

a fishy-smelling odour, particularly when potassium hydroxide is added

vaginal pH >4.7

clue cells (squamous epithelial cells plastered with bacteria).

Treatment

• Flagyl 400 mg bd patient and partner for 7 days, or a 2 g single dose.

• There may be an antabuse effect with Flagyl.

• Recurrent infections are common and can be potentiated by soap and sperm, both of which are alkaline and inhibit vaginal lactobacilli. Condoms may be helpful.

CHLAMYDIA

• This is the most common cause worldwide of non-gonococcal urethritis in men.

• In women, the cervix is infected. The infection may be eliminated, may be asymptomatic, or can spread to other genital organs to cause PID. It is as common as gonococcus.

Presentation

• In men, there is mucopurulent urethral discharge and pain on urination, which may be severe. In some cases, there is a frequent need to pass urine, and also bladder pain.

• In women in whom the infection has spread, the patient is ill with fever, and has a painful and tender abdomen.

• In neonates there is red eye and mucopus in the presence of a 'cobblestone' appearance of the conjunctival epithelium.

Diagnosis

• Send endocervical and urethral swabs for culture in chlamydia (not viral) transport medium (available from the laboratory on request).

- The swab should be sent off immediately, but if this is not possible, it should be stored at 4°C.
- In men, discharge can be examined under the microscope; sediment from the urine sample can be examined microscopically after centrifugation; samples of discharge can be sent for culture.
- In neonates, pus should be removed and the underlying cells (e.g. conjunctival) sent for culture.

Treatment

- Oxytetracycline, doxycycline or minocycline plus metronidazole are used to treat women.
- Erythromycin, 500 mg qds for 7–14 days, is suitable for pregnant or lactating women.

ACTINOMYCES-LIKE ORGANISMS (ALO)

- Reported in women who have had an intrauterine contraceptive device (IUCD) for many years.
- ALO presence is related to duration of use of an IUCD. After 1 year, 1–2% of smears contain ALO, after 3 years 8–10%, and after 5 years 20%.
- It can be asymptomatic.

Presentation

- It is most commonly asymptomatic.
- Symptoms consist of pain, dyspareunia and excessive discharge.

Treatment

- If *symptomatic*, the IUCD should be removed and sent to the laboratory with an endocervical swab for culture. If symptoms persist, refer the patient to a gynaecologist.
- If *asymptomatic*, continue with the IUCD and advise the patient to return if specific symptoms arise. Repeat the smear as per routine.

OR remove the IUCD and replace it with a copper one. Repeat the smear in 3–12 months.

OR leave the IUCD *in situ* and treat the patient with penicillin. Repeat the smear after the course of treatment has ended.

- Where ALOs continue to be reported in an asymptomatic patient, an alternative form of contraception should be sought where possible.

SYPHILIS

- This is caused by the spirochaete *Treponema pallidum*.
- This disease has three stages – primary, secondary and tertiary. The tertiary stage is now rarely seen.
- All suspected cases should be referred.

Presentation

- In primary syphilis, a hard-edged ulcer, known as a chancre, is seen on the man's penis or on the woman's vulva. Lymph nodes in the groin may be swollen.
- In secondary syphilis, the affected individual feels ill and may have headaches and joint pains. There is a pale skin rash which persists for 6 weeks and then fades slowly. A few subjects develop ulcers in the mouth, vulva or anus.

Diagnosis

- Refer the patient to a genito-urinary clinic if possible.
- A sample of clear fluid taken from the centre of a cleaned chancre is examined under the microscope to detect treponemas.
- Blood tests for syphilis are negative for about 6 weeks after infection.
- If the Venereal Disease Reference Laboratory (VDRL) or *Treponema pallidum* haemagglutination (TPHA) test is positive, the FTAABS (fluorescent treponemal antibody absorption test) is used to confirm the diagnosis.

- False-positive results on the VDRL test may occur after typhoid or yellow fever immunisation, in pregnancy, in autoimmune disease (RA and SLE) and in other treponemal infections (e.g. yaws).
- The TPHA test may be used for screening instead of the VDRL test.
- The FTAABS is highly specific and remains positive for years after infection.

Treatment

- Penicillin is used for treatment.
- Follow-up blood tests for 12 months after treatment are essential.

NB If neither primary nor secondary syphilis is treated, tertiary syphilis may develop 2–20 years after infection. This is a serious condition which carries a high risk of death at an early age, and is characterised by damage to many different tissues.

GROUP B STREPTOCOCCI

- These are occasionally seen on high vaginal swabs.
- They do not require treatment.
- Coliforms and anaerobic cocci are also normal vaginal flora.

URINARY TRACT INFECTION

- Clean-catch MSU samples should be obtained from all pregnant women, children and men with symptoms of dysuria and/or frequency.
- Otherwise, MSU samples need only be taken from patients who have complicated infections, or for whom standard treatment has failed.
- Proteinuria is a poor guide to infection. Although nitrite stick tests are better, they still have a poor sensitivity (i.e. too many false-negative results).

- The criteria for UTI are two of fever, frequency, dysuria or suprapubic pain on palpation *and* dipstix positive leucocyte esterase or nitrate. Where an MSU is taken, definite infection is confirmed by $>10^5$ organisms/ml, with >100 white cells per high-power field.

- If there are >100 white cells with *no* organisms, *consider*:
  venereal disease (VD)
  malignancy
  TB
  post-irradiation
  kidney stones.

NB Catheter infections rarely require treatment unless the patient is ill. Cultures will be positive in many catheter specimens unless they were only recently catheterised (in the preceding 2–3 days).

Other organisms

STREPTOCOCCUS

- *Streptococcus pyogenes* is the most common bacterial cause of pharyngitis.

- Antistreptolysin-O (ASO) has a normal range of <200 IU/ml.

Diagnosis

- The ASO titre can confirm infection with *Streptococcus* 2–6 weeks after the organism may have disappeared.

- An ASO titre should be requested in any condition in which *Streptococcus* is thought to be responsible for the illness (e.g. arthralgia with or without haematuria, glomerulonephritis, rheumatic fever, erythema nodosum, Stevens–Johnson syndrome).

- Titres of >200 indicate possible recent streptococcal illness.

- It is ideal to detect a rise in titres over two tests separated by an interval of 2 weeks.

- A rise in titres indicates recent streptococcal illness.

NB Several other Gram-positive organisms may cause a similar rise in titres.

Treatment

- Due to the risk of bacterial endocarditis and glomerulonephritis (Lancefield Group A), more severe cases are treated with penicillin, although milder and asymptomatic cases probably do not require treatment.

TOXOPLASMOSIS

- The protozoal parasite responsible for infection is *Toxoplasma gondii.*
- In most cases, affected individuals are asymptomatic or have only subclinical or mild infection.
- Unsuspected infection in pregnancy can be passed from the mother to her unborn child in up to 50% of cases.
- This infection is of increasing importance in immunocompromised individuals.

Presentation

- In acute illness, there is pneumonia with fever, cough, generalised aches and pains, malaise, maculopapular rash and lymphadenopathy with lymphocytosis showing atypical mononuclear cells similar to those in glandular fever.
- Rarely there is jaundice and myocarditis.
- It can cause choroidoretinitis and uveitis in adults.
- Infection passed to the child *in utero* can cause encephalomyelitis, hydrocephalus, microcephaly, cerebral calcification and choroidoretinitis.
- It may present with prolonged malaise and has been associated with myalgic encephalomyelitis.

Diagnosis

- Antibodies detectable by fluorescence or dye test appear early in the disease and persist for years.
- Complement-fixing antibodies appear late and decline more quickly.
- Around 20–40% of normal adults give positive Latex test at titres of 1/8–1/128.
- A titre of 1/256 can be expected in 1% of adults.
- Any titre, however low, should be regarded as indicating infection at some time in the past.
- Negative results are uncommon, and are therefore useful in excluding the disease.
- Antibodies may not be detectable in ocular toxoplasmosis. In ocular toxoplasmosis, some cases may give titres of *c*. 1/256, but the majority of them are in the range 1/8–1/128.
- In pregnancy, IgM determination can be useful for detecting recent infection.

Treatment

- Usually only treated in immunosuppressed individuals.
- Sulphonamide, 1 g qds, and pyrimethamine, 25 mg daily for 2 weeks, are used in all active cases.
- Supplements of folic acid are required.
- Tetracycline, 250 mg qds for 4 weeks, should be given if the above treatment fails.
- For uveitis and choroidoretinitis, use corticosteroids.
- Clindamycin is a newer alternative.

Cerebrospinal fluid (CSF)

- Normal range (mm^3): <5 lymphocyte cells.
  RBCs or WBCs (10^6/l): <1

(g/l): 0.1–0.5 protein
(mmol/1): 2.1–4.5 glucose (or no higher than
          60% of blood sugar)
Culture: no growth.

- The sample (5 ml) is divided into three tubes, one containing fluoride for glucose estimation.

Abnormal test results

- 10^3–10^4 mm polymorphs predominant, protein up to 3 and lowered blood sugar suggests bacterial infection.

- Up to 4000 cells, lymphocytes predominant, protein raised to 1–6 and blood sugar 1–4 mmol/1 suggests TB.

- 10–20 000 cells/mm^3, lymphocytes present, protein up to 1.5 and normal blood sugar suggests viral infection.

- Raised CSF glucose suggests:
    post-infectious encephalitis
    tumours
    uraemia
    diabetic coma.

- Lowered CSF glucose suggests:
    bacterial meningitis
    TB
    syphilis
    insulin therapy.

CSF PRESSURE

- Normal range: 70–200 mm H_2O.

Abnormal test results

- Raised values:
    viral meningitis or encephalitis
    subdural haemorrhage
    subarachnoid haemorrhage
    alcoholism.

- Very high values suggest:
  bacterial meningitis
  syphilis
  TB
  cerebral haemorrhage
  toxoplasmosis.

CSF COLOUR

- Yellow suggests:
  old haemorrhage and/or
  high protein content.
- Red suggests:
  recent haemorrhage
  traumatic tap.
- Cloudy suggests:
  high cell count.

Cerebrospinal fluid

	Pressure	Gross appearance	Cells (×10⁶/l)	Protein (g/l)	Protein (mg/100 ml)	Globulin test	Chlorides as NaCl (mmol/l)	Chlorides as NaCl (mg/100 ml)	Glucose (mmol/l)	Glucose (mg/100 ml)	Lange curve	Wassermann reaction
Normal	70–200 mm H₂O	Clear, colourless	0–8	0.1–0.45	10–45	Negative	120–128	700–750	2.5–4.7	45–85	—	—
Pyogenic meningitis	Increased	Turbid or purulent	1000–2000+ (polymorphs)	0.5–5.0	50–500	Positive	111–120	850–700	0–2.5	0–45	'Meningitic'	—
Tuberculous meningitis	Increased	Clear cobweb clot	100–300 (mostly lymphocytes)	0.5–1.0	50–100	Usually positive	86–103	500–600	0.8–2.5	15–45	Sometimes 'meningitic'	—
Acute aseptic meningitis	Increased	Clear or cloudy	50–1500 (lymphocytes)	Increased	Increased	Positive	Normal	Normal	Normal	Normal	—	—
Poliomyelitis	Increased	Clear	50–250 (polymorphs then lymphocytes)	0.5–2.0	50–200	Positive	Normal	Normal	Normal	Normal	—	—
Subarachnoid haemorrhage	Increased	Bloody, xanthochromic	Increased (lymphocytes)	0.5–1.0	50–100	—	—	—	—	—	—	—

3

FERTILITY AND PREGNANCY TESTING

Female hormone profiles

- Measurement of female hormone levels (usually on day 22 of the menstrual cycle) can indicate whether ovulation has occurred.
- FSH, LH, prolactin, testosterone and thyroid function should be measured between day 2–6 in the investigation of infertility in women with irregular menstrual cycles, i.e. <24 or >35 days.

SERUM LUTEINISING HORMONE (LH)

- Normal range (μmol/1):
  follicular phase, 0.8–9.0
  mid-cycle, ≤ 65
  luteal phase, 0.7–14.5.

Abnormal test results

- Levels are *raised* in:
  polycystic ovarian syndrome.
- Levels are *low* in:
  pituitary failure
  anorexia nervosa.

SERUM FOLLICLE-STIMULATING HORMONE (FSH)

- Normal range (IU/1):
    follicular phase, 2.5–9.7
    mid-cycle, up to 7.6–19
    luteal phase, 0.9–5.8
    post-menopause, 12–100.

Abnormal test results

- FSH levels are *raised* in:
    ovarian dysfunction (e.g. premature menopause, 15–30).

- FSH levels are *lowered* in:
    pituitary failure
    pituitary adenomas
    polycystic ovarian syndrome.

SERUM TESTOSTERONE

- Normal range in women (nmol/1):
    0.3–2.8 (pre-menopause)
    0.3–1.2 (post-menopause).

- Normal range in men:
    10–35.

In men, check the testosterone/sex hormone-binding globulin (SHBG) ratio. If it is less than 50 the patient may need testosterone.

Abnormal test result

- An LH/FSH ratio of >3:1 suggests polycystic disease.

- Raised testosterone in a female (>6 nmol/l) suggests a neoplastic cause. Other causes include:
    polycystic ovarian syndrome
    Cushing's syndrome
    hypothyroidism
    adrenogenital syndrome
    drug-induced causes (e.g. phenytoin, progesterone, diazoxide).

- When measuring plasma testosterone, the serum SHBG may also be measured (normal range in men is 10–50 nmol/1). As the level of SHBG increases, so usually does the testosterone level. If the plasma testosterone level is raised and the SHBG level remains normal, or at the lower end of the normal range, then a true excess of androgen exists, as in polycystic ovarian syndrome (which may be confirmed by ultrasound examination of the ovaries).

Free androgen index (FAI)

- $\text{FAI} = \dfrac{plasma\ testosterone}{\text{SHBG}} \times 100$

- Normal range = 1–10.

- SHBG and FAI are similar to thyroxine-binding globulin (TBG) and free thyroxine index (FT_4I) in thyroid function tests (TFTs) (*see* p. 132).

- SHBG varies with the menstrual cycle, and is raised in:
    women taking the oral contraceptive pill
    pregnancy
    hyperthyroidism.

PLASMA PROGESTERONE

- Measure plasma progesterone 7 days before onset of *next* period.

- Normal range (nmol/1):
    >30 indicates normal ovulation
    <16 indicates *no* ovulation
    16–30 repeat test
    post-menopause, 0.1–1.0.

PLASMA OESTRADIOL

- Normal range (pmol/1):
    follicular phase, 40–170
    mid-cycle, 440–1400
    luteal phase, 180–1000
    post-menopause, 35–175.

Investigations of female fertility

- LH/FSH
  within the first 5 days of menses
    high LH or high LH/FSH ratio suggestive of polycystic ovaries
    high FSH suggestive of ovarian resistance or failure
    low FSH or LH suggestive of hypothalamic dysfunction.

- Progesterone
  day 21 of a 28-day cycle (7 days before expected ovulation)
    low progesterone may imply problem with ovulation, repeat test.

- TSH
    thyroid disease can impair fertility.

- Testosterone
    high level may suggest polycystic ovaries.

- SHBG
    low may indicate polycystic ovaries.

- Prolactin
    high levels may indicate pituitary tumour.

Menopause

- Serum FSH and LH levels are both raised, whilst the plasma oestradiol level is lowered, i.e. oestradiol is in the range 100–200 pmol/l and FSH is >15–20 (often >30) IU/l.

- FSH >30 indicates permanent ovarian failure, e.g. post-menopause.

- 15–30 indicates peri-menopause.

SERUM PROLACTIN

- Normal range (mega-units/1):
    male, <20 mU/l
    female in follicular phase, <23 or up to 610 mega-units/1.

- Conditions that cause raised levels of prolactin include:
    physiological causes

pregnancy and lactation
craniopharyngioma
hypothyroidism
renal failure
stress
PCOS.

- Drugs that cause raised levels of prolactin include:
  cimetidine
  haloperidol
  methyldopa
  metoclopramide
  oestrogens
  phenothiazines
  domperidone
  antihistamines.

Abnormal test results

- Raised serum prolactin levels (>2000 mU/l) strongly suggest pituitary adenoma.
- Raised prolactin levels (<2000 mU/l) may be a finding in the following:
  gynaecomastia
  galactorrhoea
  infertility
  secondary amenorrhoea
  impotence
  dysfunctional bleeding, irregular cycle or amenorrhoea.
- Refer if levels >1000.

INVESTIGATIONS FOR HIRSUTISM

- Drugs such as cyclosporin, phenytoin and diazoxide may cause hypertrichosis, as may hypothyroidism and anorexia nervosa.
- Polycystic ovarian syndrome, Cushing's syndrome, adrenal tumours and ovarian tumours may cause hirsutism (unwanted and excessive hair growth), as may the drug danazol.

The following investigations may be appropriate.

- Serum testosterone concentration (normal range 0.3–2.8 nmol/l) >6 suggests a neoplastic cause.

- Gonadotrophins:
    FSH (normal range 2.5–19 IU/l); elevated levels are particularly important if associated with menstrual disturbance
    LH (normal range 0.8–14.5 IU/l); elevated levels suggest polycystic ovarian syndrome.

- Thyroid-stimulating hormone (TSH) (normal range 0.5–5.5 mIU/l). Thyroid function should be investigated further if TSH level is abnormal.

- A serum prolactin concentration (normal range 0–620 mU/l) of >1500 suggests pituitary microadenoma.

- Pelvic ultrasound examination will detect:
    ovarian pathology
    endometrial thickness.

- PCOS is suggested by raised testosterone, raised LH, normal FSH.

Semen analysis

- The initial investigation of male/female infertility involves assessment of the following:
    total sperm count
    sperm motility
    volume of semen.

- Two *fresh* specimens, produced at least 7 days but less than 3 months apart, should be provided in a clean glass or plastic container (not in a condom) and taken to the laboratory for analysis within 1 hour.

- Each specimen should be obtained after abstaining from intercourse for a minimum of 2 days and a maximum of 7 days.

- Normal range:
    >20 million
    30% normal forms
    50% motile
    motility, 90% after 45 min
                65% after 3 h
    volume, 2–5 ml
    pH, 7.2–7.8
    WBC, <1 million/ml.

- Sperm motility is graded, 1 being least mobile and 3 being optimum (random) motility.

- Sperm morphology is of limited value in the assessment of infertility, but where figures are quoted they should show normal morphology and viability in over 50%.

- Factors that affect the sperm count:
    warm testicles (suggest loose-fitting pants, avoiding hot baths, and weight loss where appropriate)
    smoking
    alcohol
    drugs (e.g. cimetidine, propranolol, spironolactone, sulphasalazine, anabolic steroids)
    varicocele (possibly).

ANTISPERM ANTIBODIES

- Circulating antisperm antibodies (IgG or IgM) may be sought or some specialised laboratories may detect antibodies in the seminal fluid or cervical mucus (IgA, IgG or IgM).

- Antisperm antibodies in one or both partners may account for up to 20% of cases of otherwise unexplained infertility.

- Antisperm antibodies are of doubtful significance when found in the serum alone. When present in the seminal plasma, titres of ≤1:32 are unlikely to have an adverse effect on fertility, but higher levels are likely to have such an effect.

- High antisperm antibodies: refer for IVF.

IMPOTENCE

- Organic causes of impotence may be neurological (e.g. multiple sclerosis), vascular (e.g. arteriosclerosis) or endocrine.

- The key endocrine disorders which should be considered in the investigation of impotence are:
    diabetes (*see* p. 125), 50% of men with diabetes are impotent
    hyperprolactinaemia (*see* p. 70)
    thyroid disorders (*see* p. 132).

- A low serum testosterone level can lead to impotence, but the effect on erectile function of declining testosterone with age is uncertain.

- The following drugs may cause erectile dysfunction:
    antihypertensives (e.g. thiazide diuretics, beta-blockers and angiotensin-converting enzyme (ACE) inhibitors)
    antidepressants (e.g. tricyclic antidepressants and mono-amine oxidase inhibitors (MAOIs))
    major tranquillisers (e.g. phenothiazines)
    anti-androgens (e.g. finasteride, cyproterone acetate, flut-amide)
    psychotropic drugs (e.g. alcohol, barbiturates, amphetamines and marijuana).

Pregnancy tests

- Urine pregnancy tests measure beta-human chorionic gonado-trophin (HCG).

NB Urinary HCG pregnancy tests do not work after 20 weeks' gestation, and should not be relied on to exclude pregnancy after a few months of amenorrhoea.

- The first morning specimen should be tested; if an unexpected negative result is obtained, a random sample should be tested and checked against the early morning sample.

- Specimens may be stored in a refrigerator and tested within 72 hours.

- Less than 50% of tests are positive in extrauterine (i.e. ectopic) pregnancies.

- In cases where an ectopic pregnancy is suspected, the serum HCG should be requested, which is 200 times more sensitive.

- A persistently raised serum HCG of >1000, on consecutive days, in the absence of an intrauterine pregnancy on ultrasound test is highly suggestive of an ectopic pregnancy.

- Serum HCG is checked after 48 hours and if it has not doubled this is also suggestive of an ectopic pregnancy. A rapidly falling serum HCG is strongly suggestive of a miscarriage.

- A urinary pregnancy test will detect >50 IU of beta-HCG and a serum test will detect >5 IU. Serum beta-HCG and pelvic ultrasound have a positive predictive value of over 90%.

- Serum HCG of <2 indicates that pregnancy is unlikely.

- Patients who have repeated false-positive tests should have their serum HCG levels measured in order to check for chorion carcinoma.

PREGNOSTICON

- Positive results can be expected 12 days after the first missed period, or 40 days after the start of the last one.

Rhesus blood group testing

- All rhesus-negative mothers with transfusions and/or an obstetric history associated with haemolytic disease of the new-born (HDN), such as three consecutive miscarriages at less than 20 weeks, one miscarriage/termination of pregnancy at more than 20 weeks, or a stillborn infant, jaundiced infant or unexplained neonatal death, should be tested.

- Samples are required before the 12th week, at the 28th and 36th week, and at delivery.

- Rhesus-positive women with a transfusion history also require regular samples (5-ml clotted and 5-ml anticoagulated samples are required in each case).

SCHEME FOR SAMPLING PRE- AND POSTNATALLY

- This should be performed for all known rhesus-negative women and rhesus-positive women who have a history of transfusion and/or an obstetric history associated with HDN since they were last tested.
- Sample required 6 months postnatally:
    rhesus-negative women delivered of a rhesus-positive infant.
- Sample required at next pregnancy:
    rhesus-negative women delivered of a rhesus-negative infant.
- No further samples required:
    rhesus-positive women with no transfusion or obstetric history.

Kleihauer test

- All rhesus-negative women should be tested within 24 hours of a threatencd miscarriage, miscarriage, termination of pregnancy (TOP), or after abdominal trauma which may result in the trans-placental transfer of blood cells.
- Fetal cells are looked for and a dose of anti-D administered (250 or 500 IU within 72 hours).
- Some centres now give anti-D at 28 and 36 weeks in the antenatal period, even in cases where there has been no risk of trans-placental transfer of cells.

Alpha-fetoproteins

- Alpha-fetoprotein may be measured in serum or in amniotic fluid.
- During pregnancy, measurement of serum alpha-fetoprotein is a routine screening test performed in most (but not all) centres.

- Used to detect neural-tube defects and Down's syndrome, it may also be of value in predicting twin pregnancies and intrauterine growth retardation.
- In non-pregnant patients, serum alpha-fetoprotein may also be used to monitor liver disease and gonadal cancer.

GERM CELL TUMOURS OF THE TESTIS

- Seminoma is AFP negative.
- 90% of teratomas have an elevated AFP or beta-HCG.

NORMAL SERUM VALUES IN PREGNANCY (µg/l)

- 16 weeks' gestation:
  26.5 mean
  <10–53, range
  >64, neural-tube defect is likely.
- 17 weeks' gestation:
  31 mean
  <10–62, range
  >74, neural-tube defect is likely.
- 18 weeks' gestation:
  34.5 mean
  <10–69, range
  >83, neural-tube defect is likely.

Abnormal test results

- Raised serum alpha-fetoprotein suggests open neural-tube defects or trisomy 21.

NB A detailed ultrasound scan of the fetus is the usual secondary investigation.

- Lowered serum alpha-fetoprotein may suggest Down's syndrome.
- The level of alpha-fetoprotein in the amniotic fluid falls steadily throughout pregnancy.

NORMAL RANGE FOR AMNIOTIC ALPHA-FETOPROTEIN (kU/l):

16 weeks' gestation, 8–24
18 weeks' gestation, 7–23
20 weeks' gestation, 3–16.

Abnormal test results

- Raised amniotic alpha-fetoprotein may indicate the following:
  fetal distress
  neural-tube defect
  twins.

- Lowered amniotic alpha-fetoprotein is found in Down's syndrome.

THE TRIPLE TEST

- The serum alpha-fetoprotein level, together with levels of unconjugated oestriol and HCG, is expressed as a multiple of the median level for a normal pregnancy of the same gestation. A computer-assisted interpretation of the result also takes into account the mother's age.

- Information required by the laboratory includes:
  gestational age, preferably based on a scan
  maternal weight
  previous history of neural-tube defect or Down's syndrome
  history of twin pregnancy or insulin-dependent diabetes in
     current pregnancy.

- The triple test is positive in 1 in 250 tests. This represents a 58% detection rate (for Down's syndrome) overall, or an 89% rate for mothers over the age of 37 years.

- The test is of limited value because of its low specificity and sensitivity.

SERUM ALPHA-FETOPROTEIN IN NON-PREGNANT ADULTS

Abnormal test results

- Alpha-fetoprotein levels of >500 µg/l suggests primary hepatoma.

- Alpha-fetoprotein levels of <500 µg/l suggest:
  primary or secondary hepatoma
  cirrhosis
  hepatitis
  cancer of the gastrointestinal tract
  cancer of the ovaries or testicles.

PLASMA OESTRIOLS (DURING PREGNANCY)

- Normal range (nmol/l):
  32 weeks, 145–800
  34 weeks, 170–1040
  36 weeks, 230–1400
  38 weeks, 300–1560
  40 weeks, 350–1600.

- Single tests are of little value, but a trend such as falling levels is indicative of fetal distress. Levels should rise during pregnancy, and therefore the absence of such an increase should indicate the possibility of fetal distress.

- Steroids and ampicillin can depress plasma oestriol values.

4

RHEUMATOLOGY

Testing for rheumatoid arthritis (RA)

The following tests may be of diagnostic help in distinguishing the many forms of RA.

ESR

See p. 15.

PLASMA VISCOSITY

See p. 14.

C-REACTIVE PROTEIN

See pp. 16 and 85.

RA LATEX TEST

- This uses latex beads coated with altered human immunoglobulin, and is significant at a titre of 1:40 or more.
- The test is negative in 20–25% of patients, especially in the early stages of the disease.

ROSE–WAALER TEST

- This uses sheep red cells coated with rabbit immunoglobulin, and is positive at a titre of 1:32 or more (i.e. 1:64 is significant, whereas 1:16 is not).

- The rheumatoid arthritis haemagglutination assay (RAHA) test has replaced the Rose–Waaler test for RA in many laboratories.

RHEUMATOID FACTORS

- Rheumatoid factor is an IgM immunoglobulin.
- Patients with early RA often have a negative rheumatoid factor.
- The diagnosis of RA should be made on clinical grounds, not just on the basis of a blood test.
- About 80% of patients with RA will develop a positive test for IgM rheumatoid factor.
- About 10% of the elderly population have a positive titre with no evidence of inflammatory joint disease.
- A RAHA titre of 1:80 is equivalent to a Rose–Waaler (SCAT/ DAT) titre of 1:16.
- The RAHA test is positive in 80% of rheumatoid patients.
- There is a false-positive rate of 5% in the normal population.

Test results

- A titre of 1:80 is weakly positive.
- A titre of 1:160 is significant.

Differential diagnosis

- If a patient with suspected RA is sero-negative (i.e. negative RAHA), obtain further information from X-rays, where RA may be distinguished from psoriasis and osteoarthritis (OA) once disease has been present for 1–2 years.
- Rheumatoid factors (usually at lower levels) can be found less frequently in other connective tissue diseases (e.g. lupus, chronic infective endocarditis and TB).

- Successful treatment of RA may result in a fall in IgM rheumatoid factor, leading to decreasing titres.

ANTINUCLEAR ANTIBODIES (ANAs)

- These are indicated in the investigation of suspected 'connective tissue disease'.
- Normal range (IU/ml) is 0–25 (titre 0:10).
- ANAs are probably best reserved for young women with features suggestive of SLE or inflammatory arthritis.

Differential diagnosis

- ANAs may be particularly useful in the differential diagnosis of peripheral symmetrical arthritis.

Test results

- In RA, the presence of ANAs strongly suggests:
    Felty's syndrome
    Sjögren's syndrome.
- ANAs are present in 20–40% of patients with RA, but are more a pointer to other connective tissue disorders such as:
    SLE
    juvenile chronic arthritis
    Sjögren's syndrome
    fibrosing alveolitis
    viral infections (EBV, CMV)
    uveitis
    chronic liver disease
    pneumoconioses
    drug reactions
    relatives of patients with SLE.

NB The incidence of ANAs in the healthy population increases with age, and false-positive tests and weakly positive tests (e.g. 1:20) are common and usually of little clinical significance.

- The frequency of low-titre ANAs in normal individuals rises with increasing age.

DNA ANTIBODY

- This occurs in connective tissue disorders, and may help to distinguish drug-induced disorders (e.g. drug-induced lupus).

COMPLEMENT

- Single-point measurements of complement are of limited value; serial levels are much more useful.

- Normal range (g/l);
    plasma C_3, 0.63–1.70
    plasma C_4, 0.11–0.45.

Test results

- Raised C_3 and normal C_4 indicates an acute-phase response (e.g. RA).

- Low C_3 and/or C_4 suggests immune-complex-mediated disease (e.g. glomerulonephritis due to immune-complex disease) or complement activation, and may be found in:
    SLE (during relapse)
    RA
    other connective tissue disorders
    cirrhosis
    pneumococcal infection
    gonococci infection
    post-splenectomy.

- Decreased C_3 in the presence of normal C_4 is seen in Gram-negative septicaemia and membranoproliferative glomerulonephritis.

- Normal or raised C_4 occurs in RA.

- In hereditary angioedema, C_4 levels are decreased during attacks whilst C_3 levels remain normal.

C_{3d}

This degradation product of C_3 is elevated in conditions that cause complement activation, and is useful for monitoring diseases such as RA and SLE.

C_1 esterase inhibitor (C_{1EI})

Low levels (30–50% of normal) are found in 85% of patients with congenital hereditary angioedema.

C-reactive protein (CRP)

CRP is an acute-phase protein, which is elevated in acute inflammatory conditions, including bacterial infections, tissue damage and inflammation.

CRP can be useful in differentiating between bacterial and viral infection and between SLE activity and intercurrent infection, as well as for monitoring RA and Wegener's granulomatosis.

- It is a non-specific test indicating:
     tissue inflammation
     damage
     necrosis
     organic disease.
- It is more sensitive than ESR.
- It is useful for monitoring the activity of RA.
- Normal range (mg/1), 0–8
     mild inflammation/viral infection, up to 40
     active inflammation/bacterial infection, 40–200
     serious bacterial infection, up to 500.
- CRP may be raised in RA and in malignancy when ESR remains normal (*see also* p. 16).

HLA–27 (HUMAN LEUCOCYTE ANTIGEN)

Test results

- This is a positive test in:
     ankylosing spondylitis

Reiter's disease
juvenile chronic polyarthritis
post-infection arthritis
inflammatory bowel disease
acute anterior uveitis
5% of the normal population.

LUPUS ERYTHEMATOSUS (LE) CELLS

• Normal leucocytes, incubated with the serum of a patient with SLE, from a homogeneous mass of nuclear material known as the LE cell.

• This test is usually only performed after a positive ANA.

Test results

• This is a positive test in:
SLE
scleroderma
chronic active hepatitis
10% of patients with RA.

Autoantibodies

The autoantibody screen usually includes antinuclear, antithyroid, antimitochondrial, antigastric parietal cell and anti-smooth muscle autoantibodies.

Antinuclear antibodies

See p. 83.

Antithyroid antibodies

Elevated titres of antithyroid microsomal antibodies with or without elevated titres of anti-thyroglobulin antibodies are found in primary myxoedema, Hashimoto's thyroiditis and Graves' disease. Elevated titres may precede overt clinical thyroid disease, and serial TFTs should be performed.

Antimitochondrial antibodies

High titres occur in 95% of patients with primary biliary cirrhosis, but low titres may also be found in patients with chronic active hepatitis.

Antigastric parietal antibodies

Antigastric parietal antibodies are present in 95% of patients with pernicious anaemia, but are also present in 3% of the normal population, and the incidence rises with increasing age. Anti-intrinsic factor antibodies are also likely to be raised.

Anti-intrinsic factor antibodies

Anti-intrinsic factor antibodies are present in 75% of patients with pernicious anaemia.

Anti-smooth muscle antibodies

- High titres (>50 IgG) are associated with autoimmune chronic active hepatitis.

- Low titres may occur in viral infections, especially EBV and hepatitis A.

Antigliadin antibodies

This is a screening test for coeliac disease and dermatitis herpetiformis. Where positive results are obtained, anti-endomysial antibodies may also be assayed.

Anti-endomysial antibodies

These confirm the presence of coeliac disease and/or dermatitis herpetiformis.

Anti-glomerular basement membrane (anti-GBM) antibodies

This test is positive in 90% of patients with Goodpasture's syndrome.

Anti-islet-cell antibodies

This test is predictive of future insulin requirement in patients with non-insulin-dependent diabetes mellitus (NIDDM) and in the relatives of patients with insulin-dependent diabetes mellitus (IDDM).

Anti-acetylcholine-receptor antibodies

This test is positive in 80–90% of patients with myasthenia gravis.

Anti-skeletal muscle antibodies

These are associated with thymomatous myasthenia gravis, but they also occur in hepatitis viral infections and polymyositis.

Anti-adrenal antibodies

These are present in 60–70% of patients with idiopathic Addison's disease, and in cases of autoimmune premature ovarian failure.

Anti-cardiac muscle antibodies

These occur in some patients with Dressler's syndrome and post-cardiomyotomy syndrome.

Anti-centromere antibody

This is used in the investigation of Raynaud's phenomenon. The test is positive in 60–70% of cases of the CREST variant of scleroderma and in 20% of cases of generalised scleroderma.

Antineutrophil cytoplasmic antibodies (ANCA)

These are indicated in the investigation of vasculitis. Two patterns exist (cANCA and pANCA). cANCA is present in 90% of patients with Wegener's granuloma. pANCA is less specific, but is associated with microscopic polyarteritis.

Antiphospholipid antibodies

These are found in antiphospholipid syndrome, which is characterised by recurrent spontaneous abortion, recurrent thrombosis (arterial or venous) and thrombocytopenia. This may occur either as a syndrome or secondary to SLE (*see also* p. 33).

Antireticulin antibodies

These have high specificity (few false-positives) but low sensitivity (high false-negatives) for untreated coeliac disease.

Anti-peripheral nerve antibodies

These are found in Guillain-Barré syndrome.

Routine testing of patients receiving disease modifying anti-rheumatic drugs

Drug	Test
Penicillamine	FBC and urinary protein weekly then monthly
Azathioprine	FBC monthly
Gold	FBC and urinary protein and blood prior to each gold injection

Continued

Drug	Test
Sulphasalazine	FBC every 2 weeks LFTs before and monthly then 3-monthly after commencing drug
Methotrexate	FBC monthly, creatinine and LFTs before starting and 3-monthly
Hydroxychloroquine	Full ophthalmic examination every 3–6 months

STOP the above drugs if the following occur:

WBC $<3.5 \times 10^9/l$
Platelets $<120 \times 10^9/l$
LFTs $>3 \times$ normal range
Urinary protein $>1g/24$ hours
Microscopic haematuria on
    dipstick testing
Macrocytosis or abrupt fall in
blood count in patients on
methotrexate

ENDOMYSIAL ANTIBODIES IN COELIAC DISEASE

Coeliac disease is an enteropathy caused by permanent intolerance to dietary gluten
(in wheat, barley and rye). In genetically susceptible individuals coeliac disease may lead to:

- vitamin B_{12} deficiency

- osteoporosis

- auto-immune disease, including insulin-dependent diabetes, auto-immune thyroid disease, auto-immune liver disease and lymphoma.

Testing for anti-endomysial antibody (EMA) is the screening test of choice, though it can be negative in up to 20% of patients with coeliac disease. If the diagnosis is strongly suspected, consider requesting total IgA quantification and IgG class antibody test. Despite a negative EMA, referral for consideration of small bowel biopsy should be considered.

Serological screening tests revert back to normal when the patient is on a gluten-free diet.

ACID GLYCOPROTEIN

- Normal range 600–1200 mg/l.
- Acid glycoprotein is an acute phase protein used as a marker of inflammatory bowel disease.

5

BIOCHEMISTRY

Liver function tests (LFTs)

SERUM BILIRUBIN

- Normal range (μmol/1) is <17; total bilirubin is 3–20; indirect bilirubin is 0–14.
- Jaundice is usually only apparent with bilirubin >35.
- If serum bilirubin is elevated, check for urinary bilirubin and urobilinogen (*see* p. 95), and if LFTs are otherwise normal, ask the laboratory to specify the level of conjugated/unconjugated bilirubin (direct/indirect).
- Sample of 5–10 ml is collected in a plain tube – there should be no additives in the tube.
- Infant blood can be obtained from a heel prick, and two blood microtubes should be filled.

Precautions

- Protect the sample of blood from sunlight, as light will reduce the bilirubin content.
- To prevent haemolysis, do not shake the tube containing the blood.
- Full protective measures should be adhered to in order to avoid self-contamination.
- Stop any medication which could interfere with the bilirubin levels for 24 hours. These drugs should be entered on the laboratory investigation form.

Factors that affect laboratory results

- A high-fat meal prior to the test.
- Carrots.
- Haemolysis of the blood specimen can give inaccurate results (the tube should not be shaken).
- Sunlight and artificial light will break down the bilirubin pigments. Light exposure should therefore be avoided so that an accurate result is obtained.
- Drugs and medication.

Abnormal test results

- Raised total bilirubin suggests:
    hepatitis
    biliary stasis
    haemolysis
    resolution of large haematoma or congenital cause (*see* below).

NB Urinalysis for bilirubin, urobilinogen and bilirubin, together with the measurement of liver enzymes and, if necessary, a breakdown of bilirubin into the conjugated/unconjugated portion will usually identify the underlying pathology.

- A raised level of unconjugated bilirubin suggests:
    Gilbert's syndrome (which affects 4% of the population)
    haemolysis (which can be confirmed by lowered Hb, raised reticulocytes (>2%), reduced serum haptoglobin and increased urobilinogen present in the urine)
    postviral hepatitis
    mild chronic hepatitis
    Crigler–Najjar syndrome (>85 μmol/1).
- A raised level of conjugated bilirubin (>10) suggests obstructive jaundice which may be due to:
    liver disease
    pancreatic disease, or
    Dublin–Johnson syndrome.

URINARY BILE PIGMENTS

- Bile, which is formed mostly from conjugated bilirubin, reaches the duodenum where the intestinal bacteria convert the bilirubin to urobilinogen. Most of the urobilinogen is excreted in the faeces, a large amount is transported to the liver via the circulation where it is reprocessed to bile, and the remainder (approximately 1%) is excreted by the kidneys in the urine.

- The urobilinogen test is a very sensitive way to determine liver damage, haemolytic disease and severe infections.

- In early hepatitis, mild liver cell damage or mild toxic injury, the urine urobilinogen level will increase despite an unchanged serum bilirubin level. The urobilinogen level in severe liver damage will decrease because the liver is unable to conjugate bilirubin or produce bile.

- Urine does not normally contain unconjugated bilirubin (which is not water-soluble).

- Urobilinogen is excreted in small quantities in the urine.

Procedure

- The single urine sample should be fresh and tested immediately using a reagent dipstick which, after being dipped into the urine specimen, is compared to a colour chart.

Factors that affect laboratory results

- Bananas.

- Antibiotics which decrease the bacterial flora in the intestine.

- Certain drugs.

- pH changes in the urine. Acid urine decreases the level of urobilinogen, whilst alkaline urine increases the urobilinogen level. Urine that is allowed to stand for 30 minutes or longer may become alkaline.

- Urobilinogen levels are highest in the afternoon and evening.

Abnormal test results

- Raised urinary bilirubin and absent or decreased urobilinogen suggests obstructive jaundice.

- Normal or raised bilirubin and normal or raised urobilinogen suggests hepatocellular failure.

- Normal urinary bilirubin and raised urobilinogen suggests haemolytic jaundice (*see* p. 97).

- False-negative tests for bilirubin or urobilinogen in the urine may occur if the urine is not fresh.

- False-positive tests for urobilinogen occur in acute porphyria.

- False-positive tests for urinary bilirubin may occur if the patient is taking phenothiazines.

- False-negative tests for urinary bilirubin may occur if the patient is taking rifampicin.

- If clinical jaundice is present, the serum bilirubin level is normal and bilirubin is absent from the urine, this is due to:
  hypervitaminosis A, or
  high serum carotene levels (normal range (μmol/l) is 0.7–3.7) due to excessive ingestion of carrots or pumpkins.

INVESTIGATING ABNORMAL LFTs

- Mild elevations of transaminases are not uncommon and should be referred for further investigation if the abnormality persists.

- The following additional investigations may be helpful:

  antimitochondrial antibodies are sensitive and specific for primary biliary cirrhosis
  hepatitis serology
  ferritin is a useful screening test for haemochromatosis
  ceruloplasmin for Wilson's disease (which causes cirrhosis and a Parkinsonian-like syndrome) (uncommon over the age of 50)
  alpha-1 antitrypsin deficiency can lead to cirrhosis (as well as emphysema)
  immunoglobulins IgG raised in acute hepatitis, IgM raised in auto-immune disease
  abdominal ultrasound.

Faecal urobilinogen

- This compound gives the stool its brown colour.
- It is produced in the small intestine by the action of intestinal bacteria on bilirubin in the bile.
- The normal range (mg urobilinogen/g stool) is 75–350.

Factors that affect laboratory results

- Antibiotics which interfere with the growth of the bacteria necessary for the production of urobilinogen.

Abnormal test results

- Increased faecal urobilinogen levels are found in increased haemolysis of red blood cells.
- Decreased faecal urobilinogen levels are indicative of obstructive biliary disease (stools will be clay-coloured).

JAUNDICE

- This is usually clinically obvious when bilirubin is >35 μmol/l.
- The following points in the history may be helpful:
  prodromal flu-like illness suggests hepatitis
  sudden-onset jaundice with severe pain in an otherwise healthy individual suggests gallstones
  slow development of jaundice, in the absence of pain or with dull, central abdominal pain, anorexia and weight loss, suggests carcinoma
  previous history of hepatitis may suggest chronic active hepatitis
  previous biliary surgery may suggest the presence of stones left in the common biliary duct
  previous malignancy, especially of breast or bowel, may suggest a biliary secondary
  details of alcohol intake should be sought

members of medical and paramedical professions are at increased risk of contracting viral hepatitis

foreign travel increases the risks of contracting hepatitis A or B.

- Drugs that are contraindicated and associated with jaundice include:

  amitriptyline
  chlorpromazine and other phenothiazines
  chlorpropamide
  erythromycin
  halothane
  imipramine
  indomethacin
  isoniazid
  methyldopa
  phenelzine sulphate and other MAOIs
  oral contraceptive pill
  rifampicin
  salicylates
  sulphonamides
  testosterone (some preparations only)
  thiouracil.

ALKALINE PHOSPHATASE

- The alkaline phosphatase test is used to determine liver and bone diseases. Alkaline phosphatase is also produced by the placenta and gut.

- The liver excretes alkaline phosphatase into the bile, and with either extrahepatic or intrahepatic obstructive biliary disease the serum enzyme level is considerably increased.

- In mild liver disease (mild liver cell damage), alkaline phosphatase may be only slightly elevated. In acute liver disease, alkaline phosphatase can be markedly elevated. Once the acute phase has resolved, the alkaline phosphatase level very quickly decreases.

- The commonest forms of liver disease that give rise to a raised alkaline phosphatase are bile duct obstruction due to gallstones, pancreatic cancer, pregnancy and drugs, as well as (rarely) primary biliary cirrhosis.

- Extrahepatic causes of biliary obstruction are usually easily differentiated by an abdominal ultrasound scan.

- With bone disorders, the alkaline phosphatase level is increased because of abnormal osteoblastic (cell) activity.

- The normal range (IU/l) is 90–300 (the level is dependent on the method of assay).

- Alkaline phosphatase is decreased when the blood sample is haemolysed.

- In children, levels are two to three times higher than normal values in adults.

- During the pubertal growth spurt, levels may be even higher.

- In the third trimester of pregnancy, levels are high (two- to three-fold).

- Post-menopausal levels are raised.

- Post-bony fracture levels are raised.

- An individual's alkaline phosphatase level remains remarkably constant up to 60 years of age.

- A slightly raised alkaline phosphatase level is a common laboratory finding. If the test is repeated and the level continues to rise, further investigations should be performed.

- A raised alkaline phosphatase in isolation, with a normal gamma-glutamyl transferase (GGT), is more likely to be of bony than hepatic origin. If the serum calcium and phosphate levels are normal, osteomalacia is unlikely, as are bony metastases. Malabsorption is unlikely if both the serum calcium and haemoglobin levels are normal.

- A normal TSH makes hyperthyroidism unlikely, and a normal prostate-specific antigen (PSA) would make prostatic cancer (with or without bony metastases) unlikely.

- A normal serum calcium level makes hyperparathyroidism unlikely. Paget's disease as a cause would be detected with plain X-rays or a bone scan.

- If doubt persists about the origin of the raised alkaline phosphatase, this can be resolved by serum elecrophoresis of the isoenzymes.

Procedure

- Use a 5–10 ml sample in a plain tube.
- There are no restrictions on food or drink prior to testing.
- Drugs that elevate alkaline phosphatase may be withheld for 24 hours.
- Any drugs that the patient is taking should be included on the laboratory request form.

Factors that affect laboratory results

- Age of the patient.
- Drug interference and interaction.
- Pregnancy in the last trimester.

Abnormal test results

- Raised alkaline phosphatase may indicate:

  bone disease: osteomalacia and rickets (Ca^{2+} <2.12 mmol/l)

  primary hyperparathyroidism with bone disease (Ca^{2+} >2.65 mmol/l) or secondary hyperparathyroidism

  Paget's disease of the bone (alkaline phosphatase level very high)

  secondary carcinoma of bone (raised Ca^{2+})

  myositis ossificans, *or*

  liver disease: intra- or extrahepatic cholestasis

  space-occupying lesions (GGT is usually raised, but bilirubin may be normal),

  hepatocellular disease, *or*

  hypo- or hyperparathyroidism (*see* p. 132).

Differential diagnosis

- Measurement of GGT is usually sufficient to confirm or exclude hepatic origin or raised alkaline phosphatase.
- 5-nucleotidase or alkaline phosphatase isoenzymes may be used to confirm the origin of alkaline phosphatase.
- Raised alkaline phosphatase and raised GGT suggests hepatic origin.
- Measurement of 5-nucleotidase (normal range 3.5–11 IU/l) can confirm or exclude hepatic origin in the presence of isolated raised alkaline phosphatase.
- Raised alklaline phosphatase and raised 5-nucleotidase suggest hepatic origin.
- Normal 5-nucleotidase excludes hepatic disease.

ASPARTATE AMINOTRANSFERASE (AST) AND ALANINE AMINOTRANSFERASE (ALT)

- Normal range (IU/l):
    AST <50
    ALT <45.
- AST (previously known as serum glutamic oxalo-acetic transaminase (SGOT)) is not included in the LFT profile in some laboratories.
- AST is present in high concentrations in heart, liver, kidney, skeletal muscle and red blood cells.
- ALT (previously known as serum glutamic pyruvic transaminase (SGPT)) is present in high concentrations in the liver. It is also present in heart and skeletal muscle, but in much lower concentrations. Therefore ALT is much more specific to liver disease than is AST.
- Transaminases are usually very high in hepatocellular disease such as viral hepatitis, and are more modestly raised in chronic hepatocellular damage and obstruction.
- AST is raised in shock, whereas there is not much elevation of ALT unless liver disease is present.

- Refer patients with high ALT (e.g. >250) immediately.
- Otherwise, a moderately raised ALT is likely to be due to drugs, thyroid disease, new diabetes or heart failure.

Procedure

- Use a 5–10 ml sample in a plain tube.
- There are no restrictions on food or drink prior to testing.
- If determining cardiac enzymes, take blood sample before administering drugs to the patient.
- Any drugs that the patient is taking should be included on the laboratory request form.

Factors that affect laboratory results

- IM injections.
- Drug interference and interaction.
- Haemolysis of the specimen.

Abnormal test results

- AST levels are markedly raised after:
  MI
  cardiac surgery.
- AST levels are raised in:
  viral or toxic hepatitis
  malignancy
  some skeletal muscle diseases
  trauma.
- Raised levels of ALT (>400 IU/l) suggest:
  acute diffuse hepatocellular damage (e.g. viral hepatitis, toxic damage, ischaemia).
- ALT levels of >150 but <400 IU/l suggest:
  chronic active, protracted, viral or drug-induced hepatitis.
- ALT levels of >1000 IU/l in jaundice suggest:
  acute parenchymal disease.

- ALT levels of <100 IU/l in jaundice suggest:
  obstructive jaundice.
- ALT > AST occurs in:
  acute hepatitis
  extrahepatic obstruction.
- ALT < AST occurs in:
  cirrhosis
  intrahepatic neoplasm
  haemolytic jaundice
  alcoholic hepatitis.
- ALT is low in:
  renal failure
  vitamin B_6 deficiency.

GAMMA-GLUTAMYL TRANSFERASE (GGT)

- Normal range (IU/l):
  males up to 70
  females up to 40.
- Synthesis of GGT is stimulated by many drugs (e.g. phenytoin, phenobarbitone, primidone, alcohol and possibly some anti-depressants).
- GGT is a sensitive test for excess alcohol intake, but is not specific.

Procedure

- Use a 10 ml sample in a plain tube.
- There are no restrictions on food or drink prior to testing.

Factors that affect laboratory results

- Barbiturates (can cause a false-positive result).
- Excessive and prolonged alcohol intake.

Abnormal test results

- Raised GGT and raised MCV suggest alcohol abuse (*see* p. 105).

- Raised GGT, history of excessive alcohol intake, raised ALT and raised MCV suggest liver cell damage.

- Very high GGT (10 times normal upper limit) occurs in biliary obstruction and hepatic malignancies.

- Raised GGT and raised alkaline phosphatase (more than three times upper limit of normal) suggests cholestasis.

- Raised GGT may be due to non-specific causes (e.g. MI, cerebrovascular accident (CVA), diabetes mellitus, chronic lung disease).

- LFTs (transaminase and GGT) are also affected by lack of exercise, obesity and smoking, as well as excess alcohol intake. Elevated results may therefore occur if several of these factors coexist, even if alcohol intake is not excessive (i.e. over 21 units).

- The effect of alcohol on GGT is complex. About 50% of people who drink alcohol to excess on a regular basis will have biochemical abnormalities, whilst the other 50% will not. An individual who is not overweight and not taking anticonvulsants, but who has a persistently raised GGT (>80 IU/l), may be 'underestimating' their alcohol intake.

SERUM AMYLASE

- Normal range (IU/l) is 70–300 (depending on the method used).

Abnormal test results

- In the appropriate clinical situation, with upper abdominal pain, vomiting and abdominal tenderness, values of >1200 are diagnostic of acute pancreatitis.

- Values in the range 300–1200 may occur in:
  perforated duodenal ulcer
  aortic aneurysm
  mesenteric vascular occlusion
  small-bowel obstruction
  ectopic pregnancy
  renal failure.

DRUGS AND ABNORMAL LFTs

- Many drugs, even when used in therapeutic doses, can cause abnormal LFTs.

- These responses usually occur within the first 3 months of treatment. Clinically obvious hepatotoxicity is rare.

- LFTs should be monitored before starting treatment with potentially hepatotoxic drugs, and monthly thereafter for the first 6 months.

- Elevation of transaminase levels by up to two-fold is usually acceptable, but the drug should be withdrawn if levels rise above this.

- Abnormal LFTs due to drugs usually resolve within 3–4 weeks of withdrawal. If this does not occur, underlying liver disease is probable.

ALCOHOL ABUSE

- Alcohol abuse is suggested by:
  MCV >99 μm^3 or fl (which may or may not be associated with a megaloblastic anaemia) (MCV is raised in 60% of people with alcohol dependence)
  serum urate >520 μmol/l
  GGT:
    males, >51 IU/l
    females, >33 IU/l (GGT is raised in 80% of people with alcohol dependence)
  AST >40 IU/l;
  triglycerides (TGs) >1.8 μmol/l
  Hb:
    males, >18 (g/dl)
    females, >16.5 (g/dl)
  ALT >46 IU/l.

- Raised gamma-globulin levels suggest chronic liver disease.

ALCOHOL INTOXICATION (SERUM VOLUMES) AND ETHANOL CONCENTRATIONS

- Subclinical intoxication (g/l): 0–1.
- Gross intoxication (g/l): 2.
- Stupor (g/l): 3.
- The legal limit for blood alcohol whilst driving a motor vehicle is 80 mg%.
- The legal limit for urine alcohol whilst driving a motor vehicle is 107 mg%.

Procedure

- A 5–10 ml sample of blood is taken, using the appropriately coloured container in which there is an additive.
- Do not cleanse the site for the venepuncture with an alcohol swab. The agent used to clean the site should be thoroughly dried with a dry swab before undertaking the venepuncture.
- The request form should have the date and time of collection of the specimen written clearly on it.

Factors that affect laboratory results

- Using an alcohol swab to clean the venepuncture site can elevate serum alcohol values.
- Alcohol and drug interactions.

SERUM PROTEINS

- These are not specific to liver disease.
- They are not very sensitive.
- Normal range (g/l) is 60–80 (depending on the method used),
- Serum (or urine or CSF) electrophoresis identifies five main protein groups, namely albumin, alpha-1-, alpha-2-, beta- and gamma-globulins.

Procedure

- Use a 5–10 ml sample of venous blood in a plain tube.
- Prevent the blood sample from haemolysing.
- The patient should not eat for at least 8 hours prior to the test. Water may be taken, and there are no restrictions on medication.
- A high-fat diet should be avoided for at least 24 hours before the sample is taken.

Factors that affect laboratory results

- Haemolysis of the blood sample.
- A high-fat diet before the test.
- Eating within 8 hours of the test.

ALBUMIN

- Normal range (g/l) is 30–55 (depending on the method used).

Abnormal test results

- Elevated albumin levels (rare) suggest dehydration.
- If albumin levels are lowered, check for protcinuria (e.g. nephrotic syndrome, malabsorption, chronic liver disease, pre-eclampsia). Albumin levels are normally lowered during the third trimester of pregnancy.

NB If albumin levels are reduced, some drugs which are usually protein-bound (e.g. phenytoin, phenobarbitone, theophylline, salicylates, penicillin, sulphonamides and warfarin), will be present in higher concentration in their free forms in the bloodstream. Therefore toxicity may be apparent at lower drug concentrations.

GLOBULINS

- Normal range (g/l) is 16–37.
- Globulins can be separated by electrophoresis into alpha-, beta- and gamma-globulins, although they are rarely quantified.

- All gamma-globulins are immunoglobulins; IgG represents 75% of the total.

Abnormal test results

- Lowered total globulins suggest immunodeficiency syndromes.
- Elevated total globulins suggest paraproteinaemias (e.g. myeloma or chronic liver disease).
- Raised alpha-1-globulin suggests:
    tissue damage (e.g. chronic inflammatory conditions and malignancy)
    oestrogen therapy.
- Lowered alpha-1-globulin suggests nephrotic syndrome.
- Raised alpha-2-globulin may suggest:
    acute inflammatory response
    nephrotic syndrome (together with lowered albumin and lowered gamma-globulin)
    diabetes mellitus
    malignancy
    cirrhosis.
- Lowered alpha-2-globulin and lowered albumin suggests:
    liver disease, *or*
    malabsorption.
- Haptoglobin is an alpha-2-globulin which is increased in acute inflammatory conditions and decreased in haemolysis.

- Increased beta-globulin suggests:
    biliary obstruction
    nephrotic syndrome
    iron deficiency
    pregnancy
    oral contraceptive pill.

GAMMA-GLOBULINS

- Normal range (g/l) (in adults):
    IgA, 1.5-2.5
    IgG, 8–18
    IgM, 0.4–2.9.

- Gamma globulins are all antibodies, and raised levels generally occur in:
    chronic infection
    RA (also raised alpha-2)
    SLE
    liver disease
    sarcoidosis.

- Gamma-globulins are commonly requested in patients presenting with recurrent chest infections or recurrent herpes infections, and in children in whom immunodeficiency is suspected.

Procedure

- Collect 5–10 ml of venous blood in a plain bottle.

- Record on the request form whether the patient has received any vaccination or immunisation (including toxoid) within the last 6 months.

- Also record on the request form whether the patient has received:
    blood transfusion
    gamma-globulin
    tetanus injection
    anti-tetanus injection.

- There are no food or drink restrictions.

Factors that affect laboratory results

- Immunisations, vaccinations and toxoids administered within the last 6 months.

- Blood transfusions, tetanus, anti-tetanus and gamma-globulin received in the last 6 months can affect the Ig result.

Abnormal test results

- Elevated IgM suggests:
    primary biliary cirrhosis or chronic infection

RA (the IgM rheumatoid factor is positive in 80% of patients with RA. The majority of the remaining 20% have IgG and IgA rheumatoid factors, but do not show up in the standard test for rheumatoid factor).

- Antimicrobial antibodies should also be sought in primary biliary cirrhosis.

NB IgM is the first immunoglobulin to appear in hepatitis A or B.

- Elevated IgA suggests:
  cirrhosis – alcoholic and other forms
  chronic infection
  autoimmune disease.

- IgA deficiency is associated with mild recurrent respiratory tract infections and intestinal disease.

- Elevated IgG suggests:
  liver disease
  autoimmune disease
  infections.

- Decreased IgG suggests nephrotic syndrome (also lowered alpha-2-globulin and lowered albumin).

- A homogeneous band of IgG, IgM or IgA on electrophoresis usually suggests myeloma, and is usually accompanied by ESR > 100.

IgE

- The normal range for non-atopic adults in the UK (kU/l) is 1–180.

BENCE–JONES PROTEIN

- This does not react with Albustix.
- It is found in the urine of 50% of patients with myeloma.

CSF ELECTROPHORESIS

- This may be useful for supporting a diagnosis of multiple sclerosis suggested by raised gamma-globulin and oligoclonal band not mirrored in serum.

Urea and electrolytes

BLOOD UREA

- The normal range is up to 8.5 mmol/1.
- Blood urea and creatinine are indicators of renal function.
- Neither plasma urea nor creatinine are very sensitive indicators of renal function.
- Urea is a product of amino acid metabolism, and is largely excreted by the kidney after filtration by the glomeruli and reabsorption by the tubules.
- Urea is therefore dependent on renal function and the rate of protein breakdown.
- It is thus elevated in hypercatabolic states (e.g. infection).
- Excretion of urea (and therefore elevation of serum urea) is decreased if vascular perfusion of the kidneys is decreased (e.g. in dehydration and congestive cardiac failure).
- Lowered urea levels occur in:
  pregnancy
  hepatic failure
  nephrosis
  diabetes insipidus.
- Raised urea levels occur in renal disease and congestive cardiac failure which is the commonest cause of a raised serum urea concentration (whilst the creatinine level is likely to be normal).

SERUM VALUES FOR UREA AND ELECTROLYTES

- Blood samples for electrolytes are best stored at room temperature, but should be sent to the laboratory within 2 hours of collection or centrifuged first.

- Blood for measurement of urea and electrolytes must be placed in the correct containers, as any contamination (even with different bottle lids) may cause errors.

- The following values are generally accepted as the normal range. Individual values may vary slightly from one laboratory to another.

- Normal range:
    Na^+, 135-145 mmol/l, 135–145 mEq/l
    K^+, 3.5–5.0 mmol/l, 3.5–5.0 mEq/l
    Cl^-, 95–105 mmol/l, 95–105 mEq/l
    Ca^{2+} (total), 2.1–2.65 mmol/l, 8.5–10.5 mg/100 ml
    Ca^{2+} (ionised), 1–1.25 mmol/l, 4–5 mg/100 ml
    urea, 3.0–8.8 mmol/l, 8.0–50 mg/100 ml
    creatinine, 60–120 µmol/l, 0.7–1.4 mg/100ml
    bicarbonate, 24–32 mmol/l
    lead (RBC), 0.5–1.7 µmol/l
    Cu^{2+}, 16–31 µmol/l, 110–200 µg/100 ml
    Zn^{2+}, 8–23 µmol/l, 0.05–0.15 mg/100ml
    Mg^{2+}, 0.7–1.2 mmol/l, 1.8–2.4 mg/100 ml
    uric acid, 0.1–0.45 mmol/1, 2–7 mg/100 ml.

ELECTROLYTE DISTURBANCES

Sodium (Na^+)

- Normal range is 135–145 mmol/l.

- Increased Na^+ suggests:
    dehydration
    primary aldosteronism.

- Decreased Na^+ may be found in:
    diarrhoea and vomiting
    glycosuria
    heart failure (on diuretics)
    liver failure
    kidney failure (occasionally).

Factors that affect laboratory results

- A diet high in Na^+.

- Drugs (e.g. potent diuretics, antihypertensive agents, cortisone preparations).

Potassium (K^+)

- Normal range is 3.5–5.3 mmol/l.

- Increased K^+ is commonly found in renal failure, which can be exacerbated by K^+-sparing diuretics, ACE inhibitors, beta-blockers and acidosis.

- Check that the specimen has not been left standing overnight, which causes haemolysis and leakage of K^+ from cells.

NB Raised K^+ levels are also found in Addison's disease (adrenal insufficiency), diabetic acidosis and renal tubular failure.

- Decreased K^+ occurs:
    in diarrhoea and vomiting
    in response to certain drugs (e.g. non-K^+-sparing diuretics, steroids, carbenoxolone, insulin and high-dose penicillin).

NB Low K^+ levels (<3.5 mmol/l) should be avoided in patients who are taking digoxin, and in those with congestive cardiac failure (CCF) or an existing cardiac arrhythmia or chronic liver disease.

- The clinical signs of K^+ depletion include:
    muscular weakness
    intestinal atony
    increased sensitivity to digitalis
    polyuria
    polydypsia.

- ECG changes which occur as a result of low potassium include flattening and inversion of the T-wave, prominent U-waves and ST depression.

- In hypertension, particularly if symptoms of weakness, polyuria and polydypsia are present and K^+ levels are low, consider Conn's syndrome (characterised by high urinary aldosterone and low plasma renin).

- Lowered urea levels occur in:
  pregnancy
  hepatic failure
  nephrosis
  diabetes insipidus.

Creatinine

- Normal range is 60–120 mmol/l.
- Raised creatinine levels occur in acute or chronic obstruction anywhere in the urinary tract.
- Lowered creatinine levels occur in pregnancy.
- Creatinine is a more sensitive indicator of renal failure than urea.

NB Serum creatinine may indicate:
  mild renal impairment (150–300 µmol/l)
  moderate renal failure (300–700 µmol/l)
  severe renal failure (>700 µmol/l).

Creatinine and ACE inhibitors

- An important complication in the use of ACE inhibitors is deteriorating renal function and/or raised potassium.
- Atherosclerotic reno-vascular disease or renal artery stenosis causes this. The incidence of this complication is 1% in patients with isolated hypertension:
  10% in diabetes
  20% in patients with cardiovascular or cerebrovascular disease
  30% in patients with peripheral vascular disease.
- For low-risk patients, e.g. isolated hypertension, it is therefore necessary to check the creatinine and electrolyte levels 2–4 weeks after commencing an ACE inhibitor and annually thereafter. In medium-risk patients the creatinine and electrolytes should be checked at 1 week, 1 month and 6-monthly thereafter. In high-risk patients the creatinine should be checked at 2 days, 1 week, 1 month and 3-monthly intervals thereafter.

- Creatinine clearance (ml/min)= $\dfrac{140 - \text{age in years} \times \text{weight (kg)}}{72 \times \text{serum creatinine (mg/dl)}}$

NB For women, multiply the resulting value by 0.85.

Chloride (Cl⁻)

- Increased Cl⁻ occurs in:
    dehydration
    severe diarrhoea
    intestinal fistulae
    respiratory alkalosis
    primary hyperparathyroidism.

- Decreased Cl⁻ occurs in:
    vomiting
    diabetic ketosis
    renal tubular damage
    Addison's disease
    respiratory acidosis.

URATE

- Normal range (µmol/l):
    males, <420
    females, <360.

- Gout is likely when uric acid levels are >600 µmol/l with normal GFR (i.e. raised levels expected in renal failure).

Test results

- Uric acid levels are elevated in:
    gout
    psoriasis
    haemolytic anaemia
    leukaemia
    polycythaemia
    renal insufficiency
    myeloproliferative diseases (including myeloma)

hypothyroidism
obesity
excessive alcohol intake.

NB Raised uric acid levels alone do not confirm gout. The uric acid level can be normal in patients with gout, and can also be elevated while the patient remains asymptomatic. Aspiration and polarised microscopy of a joint effusion or tophus is the best diagnostic test for gout.

- Uric acid levels are elevated in 30% of patients with psoriatic arthropathy.

- Low urate levels are seen in:
    patients on uriocosuric drugs (e.g. allopurinol)
    acute hepatitis.

- Drugs that raise urate levels include:
    alcohol
    aspirin (low doses)
    cytotoxic agents
    frusemide
    pyrazinamide
    thiazides.

- Dietary constituents that may raise urate levels include:
    anchovies
    kidney
    liver
    meat extract
    sardines
    shellfish
    turkey.

NB Serum urate has been considered to be a risk factor for ischaemic heart disease (IHD), and has been associated with type IV hyperlipidaemia and hypertension.

Abnormal test results

- Decreased urate excretion in the urine occurs in:
    hypertension
    hypercalcaemia

myxoedema
renal failure.

- Increased urate production occurs in:
  haemolysis
  leukaemia
  myeloma
  polycythaemia.

Differential diagnosis

- In young patients with marked hyperuricaemia, measurement of the 24-hour urinary uric acid excretion on a low purine diet identifies stone producers.

- The relatives of such patients should also be investigated, as they are at risk of nephrolithiasis.

ACID PHOSPHATASE (TOTAL AND PROSTATIC)

- Normal range (IU/l):
  total, <7.2
  prostatic fraction, <2.2.

- Do not take the blood sample immediately following digital rectal examination.

- See also the section on PSA (p. 150).

Urine biochemistry

COLLECTION OF TIMED URINE SPECIMENS

- The accuracy of creatinine clearance and 24-hour urine results depends largely on the accuracy of the urine collection. This may be difficult to control for a variety of reasons, but errors often occur because of a misunderstanding by the doctor, nurse or patient with regard to the procedure for collecting the urine. Urine already in the bladder at the time of the start of the test must not be included in the collection. The procedure is as follows for a 24-hour urine collection required between 9.00 am on Monday and 9.00 am on Tuesday.

9.00 am on Monday: empty bladder completely and *discard this specimen*.

Then collect all urine passed until:

9.00 am Tuesday: empty bladder completely and *add this specimen* to the collection.

- The components in a urine sample must be analysed within 1 hour of collection.

17-OXOSTEROIDS (17-KETOSTEROIDS)

- Normal range (μmol/24 hours):
    males 19–50 years, 28–76
    females 19–50 years, 21–52
    males >50 years, 17–63
    females > 50 years, 10–31.

Abnormal test results

- 17-Oxosteroids are raised in Cushing's syndrome.

- 17-Oxosteroids are lowered in:
    Addison's disease
    hypopituitarism.

17-OXYGENIC STEROIDS (17-HYDROXYCORTICOSTEROIDS)

- Normal range (μmol/24 hours):
    males 19–50 years, 28–70
    females 19–50 years 21–63
    males >50 years, 17–52
    females > 50 years, 10–31.

Abnormal test results

- 17-Oxygenic steroids are raised in Cushing's syndrome.

- 17-Oxygenic steroids are lowered in:

Addison's disease
hypopituitarism.

URINARY FREE CORTISOL

- Normal range (nmol/24 hours):
  males, <270
  females, <260.

Abnormal test results

- Elevation of these levels suggests:
  Cushing's syndrome (pituitary, adrenal or iatrogenic)
  polycystic ovaries
  some testicular cancers
  adrenogenital syndrome.

- Random serum cortisol levels are of no help in the diagnosis of Cushing's syndrome, which is confirmed by a raised urinary free cortisol concentration. It is essential that a complete 24-hour collection of urine is made (*see* p. 117). There is a false-positive and false-negative rate of approximately 5%.

- A low morning serum cortisol level (<50 nmol/l) after taking 1 mg of dexamethasone at midnight the previous night usually excludes Cushing's syndrome. False-positive results can be seen in:
  pregnant women
  alcoholics
  obese individuals.

- Some drugs may also influence the results (e.g. oestrogens and anticonvulsants). False-negative results are rare (approximately 2% of cases).

URINARY FREE CATECHOLAMINES

- 24-hour urine collection:
  Noradrenaline, 60–850 nmol/24 hours
  Adrenaline, up to 190 nmol/24 hours
  Dopamine, up to 366 nmol/24 hours.

- 24-hour creatinine is often quoted as a guide to the reliability of the result. If the creatinine is low this indicates too small a collection of urine took place and may invalidate the test result. Normal 24-hour urine creatinine 8800–17000 µmol/l.

VANILLYLMANDELIC ACID (VMA)

- A 24-hour urine collection is required. Add 50 ml of 20% hydrochloric acid (HCl) to the container before starting the collection. Collect three samples over 5 days. Include details of medication, especially aspirin and methyldopa.
- VMA is a metabolite of adrenaline and noradrenaline.
- Normal range (µmol/24 hours) is <36 (1.8–7.1 mg/24 hours).

Abnormal test results

- Raised VMA suggests:
  phaeochromocytoma
  neuroblastoma.

NB VMA may also be raised due to high dietary intake of caffeine, salicylate or bananas.

HOMOVANILLIC ACID (HVA)

- A 24-hour collection is required. Add 50 ml of 20% HCl to the container before starting the collection. Collect three samples over 5 days. Include details of medication, especially aspirin and methyldopa.
- Normal range (adults) (µmol/24 hours) is <42.

Abnormal test results

- Raised HVA suggests:
  phaeochromocytoma
  neuroblastoma.

NB Other features of phaeochromocytoma include severe hypertension, mild hyperkalaemia, raised haematocrit and impaired glucose tolerance.

Excretion of metabolites over 24 hours

	Mean		Range	
	SI unit	*Traditional unit*	*SI unit*	*Traditional unit*
Calcium	5.75 mmol	11.5 mEq	3.25–8.25 mmol	6.5–16.5 mEq
Chloride				
Men	184 mmol	184 mEq	120–140 mmol	120–140 mEq
Women	132 mmol	132 mEq		
Creatine			Up to 380 mmol	Up to 50 mg
Creatinine				
Men	15.8 mmol	1.8 g	9.7–23.0 mmol	1.1–2.5 g
Women	10.3 mmol	1.17 g	9.0–11.7 mmol	1.0–1.3 g
Magnesium	5.3 mmol	10.5 mEq	2.5–8.0 mmol	5.0–16 mEq
Nitrogen (total)	0.8 mmol	11.5 g	0.5–1.2 mmol	7–16 g
Oxosteroids				
Men	71 µmol	20.5 mg	59–83 µmol	17–24 mg
Women	49 µmol	14 mg	28–70 µmol	8–20 mg
Phosphate	44 mmol	1.4 g	25–62 mmol	0.8–2.0 g
Potassium				
Men	57 mmol	57 mEq	35–80 mmol	35–80 mEq
Women	47 mmol	47 mEq		
Protein		100 mg		
Sodium				
Men	177 mmol	177 mEq	120–220 mmol	120–220 mEq
Women	128 mmol	128 mEq		
Urate	3.2 mmol	0.5 g	0.5–5.9 mmol	0.1–1.0 g
Urea	342 mmol	20.6 g	209–475 mmol	12.6–28.6 g

5-HYDROXYINDOLE ACETIC ACID (5HIAA)

- Normal range (μmol/24 hours) is <31(2–10 mg/24 hours).

- 5HIAA is a tryptophan metabolite.

Abnormal test results

- 5HIAA levels are raised in:
  carcinoid syndrome
  malabsorption, especially sprue and gluten intolerance.

SERUM ALDOSTERONE

- Normal range (pg/ml):
  early morning (recumbent), 12–150
  daytime (ambulatory), 70–350.

- It is useful in testing for Conn's syndrome.

CALCIUM (Ca^{2+})

- Serum Ca^{2+} is a balance between Ca^{2+} absorption and renal excretion, bone resorption and bone mineralisation.

- Serum Ca^{2+} is usually expressed as protein (albumin) adjusted values, as it is about 50% bound.

Hypercalcaemia

- Symptoms due to hypercalcaemia are not usually apparent until the serum Ca^{2+} is >3.0 mmol/l, when anorexia, nausea, vomiting, constipation, fatigue, weakness, depression, polyuria, polydypsia, renal colic and pancreatitis may be features.

- At >3.7 mmol/l, cardiac complications can be fatal.

- At levels of up to 4 mmol/l, tiredness, malaise, lack of concentration and poor memory may become apparent, and at levels of >4 mmol/l symptoms may include nausea, vomiting, dehydration, pruritus and renal malfunction.

- The main causes of hypercalcaemia are:
  primary hyperparathyroidism
  malignancy
  sarcoidosis
  myeloma.

Abnormal test results

- Ca^{2+} >2.65 mmol/l, or >2.70 mmol/l in women over 70 years of age suggests hypercalcaemia.

- Hypercalcaemia can be due to:
  primary hyperparathyroidism (phosphate is usually <0.75 mmol/l)
  sarcoidosis
  malignancies (e.g. bronchus, breast, genito-urinary system, squamous carcinoma of head, neck or oesophagus, multiple myeloma, lymphoma)
  Addison's disease
  metastatic bone disease
  vitamin D excess or hypersensitivity
  renal tubular acidosis
  Hodgkin's disease
  Paget's disease
  osteolytic tumours or (rarely) osteoporosis
  thiazide diuretics.

- Ca^{2+} <2.12 mmol/l suggests hypocalcaemia.

- Hypocalcaemia can be due to:
  hypoparathyroidism (raised phosphate)
  rickets
  osteomalacia
  chronic renal failure
  malabsorption
  nephrotic syndrome.

- Clinical situations in which hypercalcaemia should be considered include:
  renal stones
  sarcoidosis

toxic confusional states
renal failure (may cause hypocalcaemia)
patients taking large doses of vitamin D.

PHOSPHATE

- Levels of phosphate are closely linked to those of Ca^{2+}.
- Normal range (mmol/l) is 0.8–1.45.

Procedure

- The patient may drink water and take their medication as usual.
- The patient should not eat for at least 8 hours before the blood sample is taken.
- The patient should not eat food with a high fat content for at least 24 hours before the test.

Factors that affect laboratory results

- A diet high in fat.

Abnormal test results

- Raised phosphate levels suggest:
  renal failure
  hypoparathyroidism
  vitamin D excess.
- Lowered phosphate levels suggest:
  hyperparathyroidism
  rickets (except in renal failure)
  vitamin D deficiency
  renal tubular disease
  bacterial septicaemia
  insulin therapy.

NB Drugs that can lower phosphate levels include aluminium hydroxide, anabolic steroids, oestrogen therapy and IV infusions (see also alkaline phosphatase, LFTs, p. 98).

Differential diagnosis in bone disease

- Very high alkaline phosphatase and raised Ca^{2+} suggests Paget's disease.

- Low or normal Ca^{2+} and low phosphate suggests:
    rickets
    osteomalacia.

- High Ca^{2+}, low phosphate, possible raised alkaline phosphatase and 'pepperpot' skull on X-ray suggests hyperparathyroidism.

NB With osteoporosis there are no biochemical changes, i.e. serum Ca^{2+} (when corrected for serum albumin) and bony alkaline phosphatase are usually normal.

Investigations for suspected primary hyperparathyroidism

- Fasting serum Ca^{2+} on 3 consecutive days, without the use of a tourniquet.

- Ca^{2+} excretion in the urine.

- Plasma phosphate.

- Parathyroid hormone assay, using a plastic syringe and plastic heparinised tube kept on ice, and centrifuging the sample immediately.

- Plain X-ray of hands and skull may show subperiosteal erosions and 'pepperpot' skull.

Blood sugar

- Normal range (mmol/l):
    fasting, 3.5–5.5 (may be higher in the elderly);
    post-prandial, up to 7.7.

- Use fluoride oxalate tubes for collection only, and store specimens in a refrigerator if there is a delay in reaching the laboratory.

- Glucose homoeostasis varies with age, sex, time of day and stage of the menstrual cycle in women.

- A *fasting* venous plasma glucose of 6.0 mmol/l or lower excludes the diagnosis of diabetes.

- A *fasting* venous plasma glucose of 6.1–6.9 mmol/l suggests *impaired glucose tolerance*, with an increased risk of developing diabetes, and a 40% greater risk of death from cardiovascular disease than people with a normal glucose tolerance. An oral glucose tolerance test is therefore recommended with periodic monitoring of blood glucose levels.

- A *fasting* venous plasma glucose of >6.9 mmol/l, with symptoms of diabetes (polyuria, polydypsia and weight loss), is diagnostic of diabetes.

- A *random, non-fasting* glucose less than 7.7 mmol/l excludes diabetes, greater than 7.8 mmol/l requires further investigation with a glucose tolerance test.

- A *random* glucose of >11 mmol/l, with symptoms of diabetes (polyuria, polydypsia and weight loss), is diagnostic of diabetes.

- Patients who have no symptoms of diabetes but have a fasting venous plasma glucose >6.9 mmol/l *and* a random venous plasma of >11.0 mmol/l have diabetes mellitus.

- Rarely, symptomatic diabetic patients may have a normal fasting blood glucose level.

MODIFIED GLUCOSE TOLERANCE TEST

- Maintain a normal diet for 2 days.
- Fast from midnight.
- At 8 am ask the patient to drink ³/₄ pint Lucozade within 10 minutes.
- At 10 am take blood for glucose analysis.

Abnormal test results

• Fasting glucose <7, 2-hour glucose >8 but <11 suggests impaired glucose tolerance. Check blood lipids in these patients.

• A 2-hour glucose <8 excludes diabetes.

• Fasting glucose >7, 2-hour glucose >11 confirms diabetes mellitus.

NB All figures quoted are for plasma; whole blood glucose figures are 15% lower.

CAUSES OF HYPO- AND HYPERGLYCAEMIA

• Diabetes

• Other causes of hyperglycaemia:
    hepatic disease
    acromegaly
    Cushing's syndrome
    pancreatitis
    phaeochromocytoma
    thyrotoxicosis
    hyperpituitarism.

• Drugs that can cause hyperglycaemia:
    thiazide diuretics, especially in combination with antihypertensives
    caffeine
    chlorpromazine
    dexamethasone, hydrocortisone
    oral contraceptives
    nicotine
    phenytoin
    prednisolone
    probenecid
    warfarin.

• Causes of hypoglycaemia:
    blood specimens transported to the laboratory in containers without preservative
    excess insulin or oral hypoglycaemic drug dosage in known diabetics

liver failure
pancreatic cell hyperplasia
post-gastrectomy dumping syndrome
renal failure
insulinoma.

- Drugs that can cause hypoglycaemia:
  alcohol
  aspirin
  barbiturates
  beta-blockers
  chlorpropamide
  glibenclamide
  insulin (overdose)
  MAOIs
  sulphonamides.

MONITORING LONG-TERM CONTROL OF DIABETES

HbA$_1$ (%)

- Guidelines:
  overtreatment, <6
  very good control, 6–8
  good control, 8–9.5
  increased therapy needed, 9.5–12
  careful monitoring and change of therapy, >12.

- During pregnancy a figure of <8.5 is the goal.

- HbA$_{1C}$
  normal, <6.5
  acceptable, 6.5–7.5
  high risk, >7.5.

- In the elderly, a figure of <11 is acceptable.

NB Local figures for these guidelines should be sought.

TARGETS FOR GOOD CONTROL OF TYPE 2 DIABETES

- HbA_{1C} < 7%
- Fasting plasma glucose   <6.0 mmol/l
- Blood pressure   <140/80 mmHg
- Total cholesterol   < 4.8 mmol/l
- HDL cholesterol   > 1.2 mmol/l
- LDL cholesterol   < 3.0 mmol/l
- Fasting triglyceride   <1.7 mmol/l

Serum fructosamine (mmol/l)

- Use of the fructosamine assay has replaced that of HbA_1 (in some laboratories) for monitoring the control of diabetes, because it is less expensive and it reflects average blood glucose levels over the preceding 2 weeks.

- Guidelines for adult diabetics:
    good control, <2.7 mmol/l (<350 mg%)
    control could be improved, 2.7–3.5 mmol/l (350–480 mg%)
    poor control, >3.5 mmol/l (>480 mg%)

NB These ranges are only correct when the albumin concentration is normal (30–45 g/l). Figures will vary between individual laboratories.

MICROALBUMINURIA

- A random urine sample, a timed 3-hour overnight or 24-hour urine collection, together with details of the total volume of urine, can detect microalbuminuria before proteinuria is detected on a dipstick.

PLASMA INSULIN

- Normal range (mIU/l):
    fasting, <19 (<0.9 µg/l)
    1 hour after 75 g of glucose, 50–130
    2 hours after 75 g of glucose, <100.

- Raised levels, in the presence of hypoglycaemia, may be due to insulinoma.

BLOOD KETONES

Exact guidelines on the interpretation and response to blood beta-hydroxybutyrate levels are not yet established but in the meantime, as a guide:

Blood ketone level	Recommendation
<0.6 mmol/l	No action required
0.6–1.5 mmol/l	Retest blood glucose and ketones in 2–4 hours
1.5–3.0 mmol/l	'At risk' of diabetic ketoacidosis
>3.0 mmol/l	Immediate emergency care of diabetes required

Creatine kinase (CK)

- This is the most sensitive enzymatic detector of acute MI in routine use.
- Three isoenzymes of CK exist – MM, BB and MB. MM and MB are present in cardiac muscle.
- Normal range (IU/l):
    males, 24–195
    females, 24–170.
- CK/MB is expressed as a percentage of total CK.

Abnormal test results

- If CK is elevated, ask the laboratory for CK/MB.
- A level of >6% CK/MB suggests MI. Request lactic dehydrogenase (LDH) if the patient presents with chest pain after 36 hours of normal values (100–500 IU/l). LDH is increased in venous stasis and haemolysis.

Differential diagnosis

- Normal CK 12–36 hours after the onset of chest pain usually excludes MI.

- Two normal CKs (one taken 12–36 hours after the onset of symptoms) usually exclude MI, but a significant rise in CK together with the electrocardiograph (ECG) changes and history may still support a diagnosis of MI.
- Raised CK and raised CK/MB ratio confirms MI.
- CK is also raised in:
    muscular dystrophy
    skeletal muscle disease and/or trauma (e.g. post-exercise, post-convulsion, post-injection, post-surgery)
    hypothyroidism
    alcoholism
    acute myositis as seen with some lipid-lowering drugs (e.g. clofibrate and HMG CoA reductase inhibitors (pravastatin and simvastatin)).

Lactic dehydrogenase (LDH)

- LDH is present in the heart, skeletal muscle, liver, kidney, brain and red blood cells.
- Five isoenzymes exist. The heart principally contains LDH_1, and the liver and skeletal muscle contain primarily LDH_4 and LDH_5.
- The normal range (IU/l) is 100–500.

Abnormal test results

- Elevated LDH suggests acute MI, if the patient's history is suggestive.
- CK is more valuable in the first 48 hours.

NB Elevation of other isoenzymes (<5% of results) occurs in haemolysis, megaloblastic anaemia, leukaemia, liver disease, hepatic congestion, renal disease, some neoplasms, pulmonary embolism, myocarditis, skeletal muscle disease and shock. They are also raised in haemolysed blood samples and following paracetamol overdose.

	Onset of rise (hours)	Peak (hours)	Duration of rise (days)
Enzyme			
CK	4–8	24–48	3–5
LDH	12–24	48–72	7–12

Thyroid function tests

- Normal range (serum values):
    total thyroxine, (T_4) 60–135 nmol/l
    tri-iodothyronine (T_3), 1.1–2.8 nmol/l
    thyroid-stimulating hormone (TSH), 0.5–5.5 mIU/l
    serum free T_4, 9.4–25 pmol/l
    thyroid peroxidase antibodies, up to 35 kU/l
    serum free T_3, 3.0–8.6 pmol/l
    thyroxine-binding globulin (TBG), 8–15 mg/l
    T_4/TBG ratio, 6:12.

Abnormal test results

- Raised serum T_4 occurs in:
    thyrotoxicosis
    oestrogen therapy and during pregnancy
    liver disease
    porphyria
    familial TBG excess
    drugs (e.g. thyroxine, amiodarone, propranolol, amphetamines, heparin).
- Lowered serum T_4 occurs in:
    myxoedema
    nephrotic syndrome
    hepatic failure (due to lowered serum albumin)
    kidney failure
    Cushing's syndrome

congenital TBG deficiency
hypopituitarism
drugs (e.g. phenytoin, NSAIDs).

- A very low TSH (<0.03) is indicative of hyperthyroidism. A TSH of 0.03–0.5 is suggestive of hyperthyroidism and indicates that full thyroid function tests are necessary.

- Low TSH suggests:
    thyrotoxicosis, *or* overtreatment with thyroxine of an under-active gland.

- Raised T_4, raised T_3 and lowered TSH suggests thyrotoxicosis.

- If the result is borderline, repeat the test in 3 months.

NB When treating thyrotoxicosis with radioactive iodine, the effect is not seen until about 6 weeks later. Following treatment with radioactive iodine, hypothyroidism often occurs.

- Lowered TSH and T_4 suggests:
    hypopituitarism
    overtreatment with thyroxine
    pituitary disease with or without hypothyroidism.

- Normal T_3 and T_4 with low TSH may suggest:
    thyrotoxicosis
    ophthalmic Graves' disease
    non-toxic diffuse goitre
    multinodular goitre.

CONSENSUS STATEMENT FOR GOOD PRACTICE: *BMJ*. 1996; 313: 539–44

- If TSH is raised but <10 mmol/l, repeat TSH measurement 3 months later and perform thyroid peroxidase (TPO) antibodies test. If TSH remains elevated but <10 mmol/l and TPO antibodies are detected (subclinical hypothyroidism), start treatment with 25 µg thyroxine and repeat the TSH measurement in 3 months.

- If TSH is >10 mmol/l, *even with a normal TPO*, thyroxine treatment is necessary.

• Hypothyroid women on thyroxine replacement therapy and on HRT or the combined oral contraceptive pill may need to increase their dose of thyroxine; they should have their thyroid function tests measured 12 weeks after commencing therapy.

Free thyroxine index (FT$_4$I)

• Normal range is 3.41–5.89, although different methods can cause variation in the results obtained.

• Not so commonly used.

• Has been superseded by the T$_4$/TBG ratio.

• In overt hypothyroidism, the FT$_4$I as well as the T$_4$ will be at the low end or below the normal range.

• Other laboratory tests in hypothyroidism may show:
 hyponatraemia
 macrocytosis with or without anaemia
 mildly abnormal LFTs
 raised CK.

• Other laboratory tests in hyperthyroidism may show:
 mild hypercalcaemia
 mildly abnormal LFTs.

• Elevated TSH is diagnostic of primary hypothyroidism.

• Raised TSH suggests:
 myxoedema
 undertreatment with thyroxine
 overtreatment with carbimazole or phenylthiouracil.

• Raised TSH (but not >10 mIU/l), normal T$_4$ and FT$_4$I:
 Perform a thyrotrophin-releasing hormone (TRH) test (*see* below), or more sensitive TSH assays may be helpful.

• Raised TSH (>30 mIU/l), low, normal or subnormal T$_4$ and FT$_4$I suggests longstanding hypothyroidism.

• Lowered T$_4$, raised TSH and lowered T$_4$/TBG ratio suggests: myxoedema. *Check for thyroid antibodies.*

Differential diagnosis

1 The TRH stimulation test can be used to determine thyroid function in borderline cases, or more sensitive TSH assays may be helpful.

- A normal TSH response to TRH excludes hyperthyroidism.

- No TSH response to TRH suggest hyperthyroidism.

- An exaggerated TSH response to TRH suggests hypothyroidism.

- This test has been superseded by TSH assays.

2 The thyrotrophin antibody (TRAb) test can be used to differentiate between Graves' disease and any other cause of hyperthyroidism.

- TRAbs are equivalent to TSH receptor antibodies.

- Around 50–80% of patients with Graves' disease have raised TRAb level.

- TRAb level >10 confirms Graves' disease.

- TRAb level <10 does not exclude Graves' disease.

- This test is used in few laboratories.

3 The total or free T_3 should be measured in patients with clinical thyrotoxicosis who have a lowered TSH but normal T_4. T_3 thyrotoxicosis is a rare problem (<5% of all patients with thyrotoxicosis), but occurs more commonly in the elderly and in patients with a pre-existing nodular goitre.

T_3 is also a better indicator of thyroid function in patients who are taking amiodarone, which interferes with the conversion of T_4 to T_3 and leads to falsely elevated T_4 results.

HAEMAGGLUTINATION TESTS FOR THYROID ANTIBODIES

- Normal range:
    microsome titre, up to 800
    colloid titre, up to 800 (also known as thyroglobulin antibodies).

Abnormal test results

- A value of >1600 suggests:
    autoimmune disease (e.g. Hashimoto's disease) (levels are often very high)
    Graves' disease
    simple myxoedema.

THYROID PEROXIDASE ANTIBODIES

- Normal range is up to 35 kU/l.

- Following an autoimmune antibody assay, if thyroid antibody staining is positive, a thyroid peroxidase antibodies test may be performed.

- A high titre indicates a need for regular thyroid function testing (*see* p. 132).

Long-acting thyroid stimulator antibody (LATS)

- This may be present in approximately 60% of patients with hyperthyroidism.

Thyroglobin antibody

- This is positive in 25% of cases of hyperthyroidism and in autoimmune thyroiditis.

Anti-microsomal thyroid antibody

- This is often present in hyperthyroidism and in chronic thyroiditis.

- It is positive in Hashimoto's thyroiditis and in some cases of Graves' disease.

Blood lipids

- Cholesterol is derived from dietary sources (a small proportion), chiefly egg yolks, offal and some seafood, but at least 50% of the body cholesterol is synthesised in the liver.

- There is a strong positive association between plasma total low-density lipoprotein (LDL) cholesterol and the risk of coronary events.

- A reduction in total cholesterol (TC) concentration of 10% will reduce the risk of CHD by 20%.

- Triglycerides (TGs) are the main dietary lipids found in dairy products and meat fat.

- An increase in LDL leads to hypercholesterolaemia, whilst an increase in very-low-density lipoprotein (VLDL) leads to hyper-triglyceridaemia.

- LDL is the major cholesterol particle in plasma, and high levels are strongly implicated in the formation of atheroma.

- Normal range (mmol/l):
    TC, <6.5 (desirable to have <5.2, *see* below)
    LDL, <3.35–4.0 (abnormal >5)
    high-density lipoprotein (HDL), males, ideally >0.9
                                                    females, ideally >1.2
    HDL cholesterol should be >20% of TC, or >0.2 (abnormal <0.2)
    TG, <2.3
    TC/HDL ratio, <4.5.

- The ideal TC level recommended by the British Hyper-lipidaemia Association is 5.2 mmol/l (about 80% of UK adults have TC levels of >5.3 mmol/l).

- Optimal TC levels vary with the age and sex of the individual:
    15–29 years: males, <6
                          females, <6.5
    30–60 years: males, <6.5
                          females, <7.

- Patients with established CHD should have a cholesterol level of ≤ 5.0 mmol/l and an LDL level of ≤ 3.0 mmol/l.

- Day-to-day variation in TC is in the range 4–14%. Laboratory variation may account for a further 3–5% difference in two consecutive samples. Desktop analysers may have a degree of error of up to 10%.

- Plasma cholesterol concentrations rise rapidly during the first 6 months of life and then remain stable throughout childhood. Cholesterol levels rise after puberty, reaching a peak in men between the ages of 50 and 60 years and in women between the ages of 60 and 70 years.

- LDL increases with age, particularly in women, whereas HDL remains constant.

- After puberty, HDL is lower in men than in women. Oestrogens lower LDL and raise HDL.

- LDL may be a better indicator of risk than total serum cholesterol, but it must be calculated from the other cholesterol levels, and calculation of LDL is not valid if serum triglyceride levels exceed 4.5 mmol/l.

- Blood lipids can be altered after any acute illness, including MI, and should not therefore be measured until 3 months after the event.

- Females with raised cholesterol levels are hypothyroid until proven otherwise, but renal and hepatic function and fasting blood glucose levels are also essential measurements.

- Cholesterol levels of >6.5 mmol/l approximately double the risk of CHD, and levels above 7.8 mmol/l treble it.

TRIGLYCERIDES

- The relationship between raised TGs and CHD is stronger in women and in younger patients, but alcohol and diet can obscure the relationship to CHD.

- TGs of >2.3 should be investigated. If TC is normal, assess other risk factors for CHD. If cholesterol levels are also elevated, look for secondary causes such as diabetes, renal disease, and diuretic or beta-blocker therapy or oral oestrogens.

- Raised TGs are now associated with an increased risk of CHD, possibly because thrombolysis is impaired (especially in females, but also in males, with a correspondingly low HDL). Very high TG levels (>5–10 mmol/l) increase the risk of pancreatitis.

SAMPLING

- Initial blood samples need not be taken in the 'fasting' state; a random sample is sufficient.

- The blood sample should be taken with minimal venous occlusion which could result in an artificially high cholesterol level.

- Haemolysis can cause a falsely elevated cholesterol.

- Cholesterol levels are affected by posture, the level being lower if the patient lies down, and may be affected by exercise immediately before sampling.

- Delay in the blood sample reaching the laboratory may result in haemolysis, which can falsely elevate total cholesterol levels.

- Fasting affects the TG level but not TC, and therefore a fasting lipid profile (including breakdown into HDL, LDL and TGs) will only be required if TC (non-fasted) is elevated.

- Rarely, the TC may be elevated due to an excess of HDL, which is cardioprotective, and does not therefore increase the risk of CHD.

- If the TC is raised, and drug therapy is required (*see* p. 143), then the TG level will influence the choice of drug therapy.

- The sample should not be taken after removal of the tourniquet.

Test results
- TC >6.5 mmol/l:
    take sample in 'fasting' state and request TGs and HDL.

- TC >6.5 mmol/l suggests hypercholesterolaemia (a significant risk factor for IHD/coronary artery disease (CAD)).

- TC 5.2–6.5 mmol/l:
    dietary advice only is required, and the test may be repeated in 1–2 years.

- TC <5.2 mmol/l:
    repeat test in 5–15 years according to the patient's age and sex.

NB Hypercholesterolaemia may be secondary to:
    diabetes mellitus
    excess alcohol intake

hypothyroidism (especially in elderly females)
biliary obstruction
chronic renal failure
hypotension
nephrotic syndrome
obesity
pregnancy
therapy with some beta-blockers, steroids, thiazide diuretics, isotretinoin and psoriatic drugs (e.g. Tigason) (always check lipids in patients with psoriasis before giving the drug).

- Up to 70% of hyperlipidaemia is due to one of the above primary disorders.

WHO SHOULD HAVE THEIR LIPIDS MEASURED?

- Patients with existing CHD, peripheral vascular disease (PVD) or cerebrovascular disease.

- Patients with a first-degree relative with CHD before the age of 55 years in men or 65 years in women.

- Patients with a family history of raised cholesterol or TG levels.

- Patients with corneal arcus before the age of 45 years or patients with xanthelasma or tendon xanthoma.

- Patients with other risk factors for CHD, such as diabetes mellitus, hypertension, smoking or obesity (BMI >30).

GENERAL PRINCIPLES OF TREATMENT OF HYPERCHOLESTEROLAEMIA

- The primary aim is to reduce lipid levels to acceptable values (6–6.5 mmol/l in the UK), primarily by a low-fat diet (<10% of total calories derived from saturated fat and <30% of total calories derived from all fat), or drug therapies (*see* p. 143) if diet fails and other risk factors are present.

- Other risk factors for IHD should also be eradicated (e.g. smoking, obesity, excess alcohol, hypertension).

NB *Never regard lipids in isolation. Always look at the patient's other CHD risk factors.*

Treatment groups

1 TC 5.2–6.5 mmol/l and TGs <2.2 mmol/l

- Lipid-lowering diet (*see* above).
- Weight control (to within 10% of target weight, *see* p. 142).
- Reduction in alcohol intake, where appropriate.
- Drugs are very rarely necessary, usually only if the HDL is very low (e.g. 0.5).
- Follow-up at 6 months if other risk factors for IHD are present; otherwise follow-up is optional.
- Patients with a history of CHD or following a CABG may benefit from more aggressive attempts, including drug therapy to reduce their cholesterol to <5.2 mmol/l.
- If there is no improvement:
  reinforce dietary advice
  consider drug therapy (depending on the overall CHD profile and HDL level).

2 TC 6.5–7.8 mmol/l and TGs < 2.2 mmol/l

- Lipid-lowering diet.
- Weight control.
- Follow-up at 2–4 months.
- If there is no improvement:
  reinforce dietary advice
  consider drug therapy (depending on the overall CHD risk profile and HDL level).

- More aggressive therapy may benefit patients with multiple risk factors for CHD.

3 TC <5.2 mmol/l and TGs 2.3–5.6 mmol/l

- Lipid-lowering diet.
- Weight control (including alcohol).

- Drug therapy.
- Follow-up at 12 months; assess efficacy of drugs.
- If there is no improvement:
  reinforce dietary advice
  reassess in 6 months if other risk factors for IHD are present.
- If there is improvement, reassess in 1–5 years.

4 TC 5.2–7.8 mmol/l and TGs 2.3–5.6 mmol/l

- Lipid-lowering diet.
- Weight control.
- Follow-up at 2–4 months.
- If there is no improvement:
  consider drug therapy.

NB Few patients in category 4 have primary hyperlipidaemia. Most of them are overweight, have diabetes and/or drink too much alcohol. Drug therapy may also be a factor (e.g. diuretics, beta-blockers).

5 TC >9 mmol/l or TGs >112 mmol/l may indicate rare lipid disorders (*see* p. 144), often of genetic origin, which may require precise diagnosis and initial treatment at a lipid clinic.

Dietary advice

- Reduce calorie intake in order to achieve weight control.
- Replace saturated fats (mostly animal fats) with poly- and mono-unsaturated fats (mainly vegetable and fish oils). Saturated fats raise the plasma concentration of LDL cholesterol and potentiate the hypercholesterolaemic effect of dietary cholesterol.
- Increase intake of fresh vegetables, fruit, wholemeal bread, fibre, oats and pulses.

NB Although eggs are high in cholesterol, they are not high in total fat, and therefore up to 6 eggs per week may be included in a total low-fat diet. If cholesterol levels are very high, a diet free from eggs or with a maximum of 3 eggs per week should be advised.

- Consider referral to a dietitian.
- Drug therapy.

Drug treatment of hyperlipidaemias

- Drugs that lower lipid levels may be considered in:
  - subjects with known vascular disease, when diet alone has failed
  - subjects with familial hypercholesterolaemia
  - subjects with a family history of IHD/CHD
  - subjects whose cholesterol level is >7.8 mmol/l, and who have a high risk for CHD and seem to have a primary lipidaemia, especially where the HDL ratio is <0.2 (or <20% of the TC). Many post-menopausal women have a high HDL and, despite a high TC, may not require treatment at all.
- Agents include:
  - bezafibrate/gemfibrozil (not very effective in patients with pure hypercholesterolaemia, but the agents of choice in mixed hyperlipidaemia)
  - colestipol/cholestyramine (the first choice for pure hypercholesterolaemia)
  - simvastatin/pravastatin (best reserved for familial hypercholesterolaemia or for those who have failed on other drugs, although their application is now widening with lipidaemia).
- Maxepa decreases TC in some patients, decreases TGs and raises HDL.
- Drugs which may adversely affect blood lipids include:
  - some diuretics (including thiazides, loop diuretics and K+-sparing diuretics)
  - some beta-blockers (except for pindolol, acebutolol and labetol)
  - norgestrel-containing oral contraceptives
  - isotretinoin (for treatment of acne)
  - Tigason (for treatment of psoriasis).

RARE LIPID DISORDERS

Familial hypercholesterolaemia

- There are two forms of this inherited condition:
  heterozygous familial hypercholesterolaemia
  homozygous familial hypercholesterolaemia (very rare, approximately 1 in 1 million births).

- Features include:
  TC >6.7 mmol/l, sometimes >9 mmol/l (average about 10.5 mmol/l)
  LDL elevated 2–10 times above normal
  normal TG levels
  tendon xanthomas about the knee, elbow and the dorsum of the hand
  xanthelasma
  corneal arcus
  family history of early CHD and MI or xanthomas.

- Treatment involves:
  lipid-lowering diet
  limiting other risk factors
  drug therapy (e.g. Questran, simvastatin, pravastatin)
  plasma exchange in severe cases.

Familial triglyceridaemia

- Features (not usually exhibited until puberty/early adulthood) include:
  TG levels >2.5 mmol/l
  VLDL levels elevated.

- Affected individuals frequently have the following characteristics:
  obesity
  hyperglycaemia
  hyperinsulinaemia
  hypertension
  hyperuricaemia
  excess acohol intake.

- If the levels of chylomicrons is increased, pancreatitis may develop.

- Treatment is as follows:
    control obesity
    restrict calories, saturated fat and alcohol intake
    avoid oral contraceptives
    treat diabetes mellitus and hypothyroidism if present
    if all of these measures fail, consider drug therapy (e.g. Maxepa).

Familial combined hyperlipidaemia

- Features include:
    elevation of TC and TG levels from puberty onwards
    lipid level increases are often mild and can change with time
    strong family history of premature CAD
    xanthomas absent.

- Treatment is as follows:
    weight reduction
    lipid-lowering diet
    avoid alcohol
    avoid oral contraceptives
    limit other risk factors
    if there is elevation of TG levels, give Maxepa.

NB Lowering the level of cholesterol pharmacologically may increase the TG level, thereby negating any benefit obtained by this manoeuvre.

Familial dysbetalipoproteinaemia

- Features include:
    elevated TC levels
    elevated TG levels
    xanthomas of palms and digital creases in about 50% of cases
    tuberous or tubero-eruptive xanthomas over the elbows and knees
    xanthelasma
    corneal arcus.

NB Clinical features are not usually manifested until the affected individual is over 20 years old.

- Patients with clinical manifestations of this condition often have the following:
    diabetes mellitus
    hypothyroidism
    obesity
    excess alcohol intake.

- Affected individuals at high risk of IHD and peripheral vascular disease manifest mainly with claudication.

- Treatment is as follows:
    treat hypothyroidism and diabetes mellitus if present
    control obesity
    lipid-lowering diet
    limit other risk factors
    if all of these measures fail, consider drug therapy (e.g. Bezalip).

FREIDRICKSON'S CLASSIFICATION OF HYPERLIPO-PROTEINAEMIA

Type I

- Cholesterol normal.
- TG greatly increased.
- Hyperchylomicronaemia.

Type IIa

- Cholesterol increased.
- LDL increased.
- TG normal.

Type IIb

- Cholesterol increased.
- VLDL increased.

- TG increased.
- LDL increased.

Type III

- Cholesterol increased.
- TG increased.
- VLDL cholesterol/VLDL TG >0.35.
- Floating betalipoproteins.

Type IV

- Cholesterol normal or increased.
- VLDL increased.
- TG increased.

Type V

- Cholesterol increased.
- LDL reduced.
- Chylomicrons and VLDL increased.
- TG greatly increased.

Special cases

HIGH TC AND HIGH HDL

- Although HDL is cardioprotective, it is not known to what extent high HDL levels continue to exert a cardioprotective effect when associated with a high TC level.

VERY HIGH TG LEVELS

- Very high TG levels (>4.5 mmol/l) may be caused by a primary metabolic defect or be secondary to alcohol, diabetes or drug therapy, especially protease inhibitors such as indinavir, nelfinavir, ritonavir and saquinavir, which are used in the treatment of HIV infection. Protease inhibitors are also associated with lipodystrophy and insulin resistance.

- The role of TGs as an independent coronary risk factor has become established, and the preferred treatment option for post-MI patients with a commonly found mixed picture of raised LDL (but <4.7 mmol/l), low HDL (<0.92 mmol/l) and a high TG level (>2.3 mmol/l) is a fibrate.

- TG concentrations of >10 mmol/l carry an increased risk of acute pancreatitis and require urgent treatment.

NB Patients with high TG levels often respond well to diet or treatment of the underlying cause, such as withdrawal of alcohol.

INHERITED HYPERLIPIDAEMIAS

- Familial hypercholesterolaemia affects 1 in 500 of the UK population.

- Heterozygotes often have a TC level of 7.5–15 mmol/l. They also often have corneal arcus or tendon xanthoma, and they require drug treatment.

- Homozygotes often have a TC level of 15–30 mmol/l. They are at very high risk of early-onset (often in early childhood) cardiovascular disease.

- Some patients will have very high TC (10–15 mmol/l) and TG levels (5–12 mmol/l). These patients often have palmar-crease xanthomas. They respond well to treatment with fibrates.

TREATMENT OF HYPERLIPIDAEMIA

- Patients with CHD, cerebrovascular disease or PVD are already at risk of further episodes. Therefore TC should be reduced to <5 mmol/l and LDL to <3.2 mmol/l.

- In patients with no past history of CHD, a calculated 10-year risk of >30% (3% per annum) is regarded as high enough to require reduction of modifiable risk factors (including blood pressure, weight, smoking and hyperlipidaemia), with drug therapy if necessary.

- The risk of CHD from smoking increases with the number of cigarettes smoked. Smokers have an increased risk of sudden cardiac death of between two- and four-fold.

- Diabetic patients have at least double the risk of MI.

Drug treatment of hyperlipidaemia

- Before commencing drug treatment to lower cholesterol and/or TGs, dietary measures such as reducing dietary cholesterol and calorie intake from saturated fat, and total calorie intake if the patient is overweight, should be instigated.

- Exercise not only helps to reduce weight and therefore the total risk of CHD, but also elevates cardioprotective HDL levels.

- Statins are the drugs that are most effective in reducing TC and LDL levels and, to a lesser extent, TGs if these are not too high (≤ 5 mmol/l).

- Fibrates are most effective in reducing serum TG levels (often by around 30–40%), but are less effective than statins in decreasing cholesterol levels. Fenofibrate also has a modest effect in reducing serum uric acid levels, which may be useful in patients with coexisting gout. The omega-3 fish oils reduce TG levels.

- Bile-acid sequestrants reduce LDL levels but cause an increase in TGs.

MONITORING STATIN THERAPY

- LFTs are required before commencing treatment with a statin.
- 3 months after commencing statin therapy measure lipids, LFTs and possibly creatine kinase.
- Repeat LFTs 6-monthly or sooner if dose of statin increased.

- Stop statin if transaminase levels are 3 × the upper limit of the normal range, or if creatine is 'significantly raised', particularly if the patient complains of muscle cramps.

PROSTATE-SPECIFIC ANTIGEN (PSA)

- Prostate cancer is the second most common cause of cancer-related death in males and is likely to overtake lung cancer as the commonest cause of cancer-related death in males within the next 5 years.

- PSA is a glycoprotein specific to prostatic tissue. It is regarded as a useful tool for monitoring the response to treatment of prostatic cancer, and as a predictor of relapse. It is also being increasingly used as a screening test. Whilst screening for prostatic cancer by measuring PSA remains controversial, an editorial in the *Lancet* suggested that 'No evidence of benefit from PSA screening is not the same as evidence of no benefit'.

- PSA is organ specific but not disease specific.

- An increase in PSA level above the normal range can be found after recent sexual activity, cycling, prostatic massage (not after digital rectal examination), transrectal ultrasound examination, urinary infection and cystoscopy.

- When the total PSA is raised, the free/total PSA ratio increases the specificity (i.e. there are fewer false-positives) of the test.

PSA age reference ranges

Age (years)	Total PSA reference range (µg/l)
40–49	0–2.5
50–59	0–3.5
60–69	0–5.0
70–79	0–6.0

- In all men with results in the range 4–9.0 µg/l, and in men under 59 years with a raised PSA (>3.5 for age 50–59 years and >2.5 for age ≤ 49 years), the free/total PSA ratio may be helpful:

>15%, malignancy is unlikely
5–15%, requires investigation
<5%, malignancy is likely.

- The % of free PSA or free/total PSA is not reliable when the total PSA >10 mg/l.

PSA velocity

- An increase of more than 25% in the PSA level within 12 months should warrant referral for possible further investigation, such as prostatic biopsy.

TESTING FOR *HELICOBACTER PYLORI*

- *Helicobacter pylori* is implicated in peptic ulceration, and its erad-ication can lead to healing of ulcers. Its relevance in non-ulcer dyspepsia is less clear.

- *H. pylori* can be detected from biopsy specimens at endoscopy, or by serology or the urea breath test. The urea breath test requires the patient to swallow a radiolabelled carbon isotope, which is exhaled as radiolabelled carbon dioxide.

- An exhaled $^{14}CO_2$ of >0.25 indicates the presence of *H. pylori*, or the failure of eradication following treatment.

- Exhaled $^{14}CO_2$ is expressed as % dose/mmol CO_2 multiplied by the patient's body weight in kilograms.

Faecal fats

- The test for fat in the stool is used to determine the malabsorp-tion syndrome. Stool specimens are collected to see if fat is being digested.

- Fat will not be digested if the patient has pancreatic disease with a deficiency of lipase, biliary obstruction or some other intestinal malabsorption condition.

- If there is steatorrhoea or excess fat in the stools, the latter will be frothy, foul-smelling, greyish and greasy. The patient will also have foul-smelling flatus.
- Normal range (mmol/24 hours):
    adults, 5–18
    children >6 years, <14.

Procedure

- Collect all stool specimens for 3 days.
- Collect the entire stool and label with the date and time.
- Weigh the specimen container prior to collection of the stool.

Factors that affect the laboratory results

- Ingestion of barium will make the test invalid for 48 hours.
- Mineral oil, laxatives and enemas will interfere with testing, and should not be administered.

Test results

- Raised levels suggest:
    malabsorption
    pancreatic disease.

Reducing substances

- Their presence in the faeces suggests malabsorption (e.g. lactase intolerance).

Coeliac disease

- Clinical features:
    iron deficiency anaemia
    weight loss

diarrhoea
abdominal pain
failure to thrive (in children).

* IgA anti-gliaden antibody level raised:
    normal, 2–90 U/l.

6

MISCELLANEOUS

Interpretation of cervical smears

This is a guide to descriptive terminology used by laboratories when reporting cervical smears. Different laboratories may use different terms, and if there is any doubt about the meaning of a report or what action should be taken, the individual laboratory should be consulted.

INFLAMMATORY CHANGES

- This is a redundant term that is no longer routinely reported and has been largely replaced by 'borderline changes' (*see* below).

Action

- Repeat the smear at least twice before returning to normal recall.

NB A negative smear with inflammatory changes does not require follow-up in the absence of the report of a specific infection, but may require further investigation if appropriate.

DYSKARIOSIS

- Changes in squamous epithelial cells, which may indicate the presence of cervical intra-epithelial neoplasia (CIN), are reported as dyskariotic and graded mild, moderate or severe (roughly equivalent to CIN 1, CIN 2 and CIN 3, respectively).

- Severe dyskariosis may be reported as abnormal squamous cells suggesting carcinoma *in situ.*

- Human papilloma virus (HPV) infection may be indistinguishable from mild dyskariosis.

Action

- Colposcopy is necessary for all moderate and severe dyskariosis, but for mild dyskariosis a single repeat smear is usually required to confirm the diagnosis.

HUMAN PAPILLOMA VIRUS (HPV) INFECTION

- Changes due to HPV are reported together with the nuclear abnormality, such as dyskariosis or borderline changes.

- If cytological evidence of HPV is present but there is no evidence of dyskariosis, then the smear is reported as borderline and the HPV changes are noted on the smear report.

Action

- The management of sub-clinical HPV infection is dependent on the degree of nuclear abnormality present, as is the recall of women with evidence of HPV on the cervical smear.

- HPV infection may mimic the changes of mild dyskariosis (e.g. at colposcopy, evidence of HPV infection may be found with no evidence of CIN).

KOILOCYTES

- These are cells with a halo around their nucleus.

- They indicate infection with HPV, which may be involved in the aetiology of CIN.

DYSKERATOSIS

- There is cornification/keratinisation of cells.

- This also indicates infection with HPV.

BORDERLINE CHANGES

- Cells cannot be described as normal.
- Changes resembling mild dyskariosis may be present.
- In patients with persistent borderline changes, this may indicate the presence of CIN.

Action

- Follow the local laboratory guidelines.
- The usual laboratory policy is to refer for colposcopy after three borderline smear reports.

GLANDULAR ABNORMALITIES

- Abnormal glandular cells in the cervical smear may arise from the endocervix or less often from the endometrium.

Action

- Refer the patient.

ACTINOMYCES OR ALOs

See p. 57.

METAPLASTIC CELLS

- These are normal cells from the transformation zone.
- Occasionally atypical metaplastic cells are observed, which are likely to be due to inflammation or HPV infection. Squamous or endocervical neoplasia is less likely.

Action

- Repeat the smear and refer the patient for colposcopy if the condition is persistent.

ABNORMAL METAPLASTIC CELLS

- These are more likely to be neoplastic, and are usually squamous rather than glandular.

Action

- Refer the patient for colposcopy.

QUALITY OF CERVICAL SMEARS

- Some laboratories comment on the quality of cervical smears.
- The perfect smear should contain endocervical cells, metaplastic cells and squamous cells, all in adequate numbers (*see* the British Society for Clinical Cytology (BSCC) guidelines below).
- Where the laboratory classifies smears as 'good', 'adequate', 'acceptable' or 'poor', a clear understanding of these terms should exist.
- 'Good' or 'adequate' indicates that there is sufficient cellular material to exclude any abnormalities requiring follow-up.
- 'Acceptable' or 'poor' will require a repeat smear sooner than 3 years, and the laboratory will usually indicate how soon this should be. An endocervical brush may be necessary for the repeat smear.
- In women using oral contraceptives, smears should be taken during the first half of the cycle, e.g. days 4–15.
- In women not using oral contraceptives, smears should be taken any time except the first 4 days.

BSCC GUIDELINES

- The transformation zone should be the prime target for cervical cytology sampling.

- The ideal smear should contain endocervical cells, metaplastic cells, endocervical mucus and squamous cells.
- Squamous cells and at least two of the other three elements should be present in an adequate smear.
- The cells on the slide should appear to be associated together in streaks rather than having the flat, rather dispersed appearance of a vaginal smear.
- The quality of this cellular material should be such that, if condensed into an area of 40×22 mm, the epithelial cells would occupy at least 25% of this area. The quality of the material is more important than the quantity.

POSTNATAL SMEAR

- Many polymorphs may be present and obscure the cells such that abnormal cells cannot be excluded.
- The smear may be affected by altered hormonal status.

Action

- The smear should be repeated.

NB A laboratory report of an apparently low oestrogen level may be made on a smear taken shortly after a pregnancy, or may indicate an endocrine abnormality or exogenous hormones.

Microscopic haematuria

- Normal rate of urinary excretion of RBC: 20 000–40 000/h.
- The urinary dipstick can detect less than 1000 cells/ml unspun urine.
- The urinary dipstick has a sensitivity of 100% but a specificity of 60%.
- It is not uncommon for asymptomatic individuals to be detected on medical screening.

- The 'normal' upper acceptable limit for the presence of red cells on microscopy has yet to be universally agreed but is between 2 and 5 erythrocytes per high power field.

- Microscopic haematuria is rare before the age of 50 (occurring in fewer than 1 in 100 people of this age); after 50 years of age the prevalence rises to between 2% and 18%.

Abnormal test results

- Asymptomatic microscopic haematuria should always be further investigated by microscopy, and culture and sensitivity.

- Some laboratories restrict the number of specimens on which they perform 'routine microscopy' but both microscopy, and culture and sensitivity are necessary in the management of asymptomatic microscopic haematuria.

- Microscopy of urine for white cells and red cells identifies evidence of inflammation for which infection is one of many causes. Other causes of inflammation in the urinary tract include ureteric stone and nephritis. Red cells may also come from a bladder tumour.

- A urine sample should be sent to the laboratory in a container with boric acid as a preservative to prevent the breakdown of the sample in transit.

- Phase contrast microscopy can identify the morphology of red blood cells, if present, and can distinguish dysmorphic cells whose origin is renal.

Diagnosis

- Microscopy of unspun urine specimen is unreliable: it fails to reveal 80% of patients with known disease.

- Centrifugation of urine increases sensitivity $\times$ 300.

- Most common non-renal tract causes of false-positive Dipstix test:
  menstruation in women
  preputial or meatal lesions in men
  following rectal examination.

- Bacterial contamination or sterilisation of the urine bottle can give false-positive result on Dipstix.
- Presence of RBC on microscopy, after centrifugation of urine, *confirms* haematuria and *excludes* false-positive Dipstix test.
- Concurrent treatment with anticoagulants *does not exclude* renal tract pathology; investigation of microscopic haematuria should still be performed.

Faecal occult blood

- A positive FOB may be indicative of any ulcerative or neoplastic disease of the GI tract, including:

  oesophageal varices
  peptic ulcer
  blood loss from the upper or lower GI tract due to drugs (e.g.
      aspirin or NSAIDs)
  inflammatory bowel disease
  haemorrhoids
  benign or malignant lesions of the bowel.

- Colorectal cancer is the third most common cancer in the UK (lung cancer, first, prostatic cancer, second), accounting for 23 000 new cases per year.
- Its frequency increases with age, the incidence doubling with each decade over 40 years.
- Two out of three people will die, whilst only 50% of newly diagnosed cases will have a lesion which can be totally cured by surgery.
- If colorectal cancer is diagnosed early, whilst restricted to the mucosa (Dukes' A), there is a 95% 5-year cure rate.
- Adenomatous polyps arising in the bowel mucosa have an increased likelihood of becoming malignant with increasing size.
- Faecal specimens should be at least 12 hours old before testing for occult blood, to allow sufficient time for haemoglobin to be converted to haematin.

- Weakly positive tests become negative within 2–4 days of storage at room temperature.

- Strongly positive stool samples still react after 10 days.

- Three stool samples, usually on consecutive days, will miss about 10% of tumours. The occult blood reaction is not specific for human haemoglobin, hence a 3-day meat-free diet is recommended prior to the test.

- Oral iron preparations can cause false positive reactions and aspirin can cause gastrointestinal bleeding which is unrelated to gut pathology. Ascorbic acid, which is an anti-oxidant, interferes with the development of the colour reaction in the test.

- The following should be excluded from the diet for 3 days before collecting the stool sample for FOB testing:
   red meat
   cauliflower
   broccoli
   turnips
   bananas
   radish.

- Most larger polyps bleed, hence the faecal occult blood test may be useful as a screening tool. The test is safe, inexpensive and non-invasive. It does however have limitations – it will only detect larger polyps or cancers. As colorectal cancers only bleed intermittently it is a relatively insensitive test and many false-negative results occur. Moreover, as other non-malignant lesions cause a positive result it is also non-specific.

- Screening of asymptomatic people >45 years reveals 2% being positive. Of these, there is a 1:10 chance of having a carcinoma, and a 1:3 chance of having an adenoma. >50% of the detected tumours are early lesions, compared with only 10% of the unscreened population.

Therapeutic target ranges of commonly monitored drugs

- Check local laboratory ranges.
- Write on request form stated time of the last dose.

	Metric units	Molar units
Aminophylline	10–15 µg/ml	
Carbamazepine	4–10 mg/l	17–42 µmol/l
Clonazepam	15–60 µg/l	60–150 nmol/l
Digoxin	0.5–2.0 ng/ml	1.0–2.6 nmol/l
(assuming normal potassium and renal function)		
Digoxin toxicity is likely at levels above 3.5 nmol/l		
Ethosuxamide	40–100 mg/l	283–708 µmol/l
Isoniazid	1–7 mg/l	
Lithium	4–11 mg/l	0.4–1.2 mmol/l
Phenobarbitone	10–40 mg/l	40–172 µmol/l
Phenytoin	10–20 mg/l	40–80 µmol/l
Primidone	5–15 mg/l	23–55 µmol/l
Procainamide	4–8 µg/ml	17–34 µmol/l
Sodium valproate	50–100 mg/l	347–693 µmol/l
Theophylline	10–20 mg/l	56–111 µmol/l

NB Digoxin toxicity is normally associated with serum levels >3 ng/ml, although it can be toxic within the therapeutic range. Many patients complain of sedation at therapeutic phenobarbitone levels of >25 mg/l (100 µmol/l).

LITHIUM CARBONATE

- Therapeutic range (mmol/l): 0.4–0.8 12-hour post-ingestion.

Precautions

- Plasma concentrations must be measured regularly (every 1–3 months on stabilised regimens).

- Thyroid function must be checked regularly and adequate sodium and fluid intake maintained.
- Urea, electrolytes, creatinine and TFTs should be measured annually unless indicated sooner.

Possible contraindications

- *Avoid* in renal impairment, cardiac disease, conditions with sodium imbalance, e.g. Addison's disease.
- *Caution* in pregnancy (fetal intoxication), breast-feeding mothers, elderly patients, myasthenia gravis and diuretic treatment.

Dosage

- Initially 0.25–2.0 g daily.
- Start with 200–500 mg lithium carbonate for the first week or two, measuring the serum lithium weekly and increasing the dose of lithium (Li^+) to between 300 and 1250 mg nocte until the serum level reaches 0.4–0.8 mmol/l (*see* below).
- Adjust to achieve plasma concentration on 0.4–0.8 mmol/l by tests on samples taken 12 hours after the preceding dose on the 4th and 7th days of treatment, then weekly until dosage has remained constant for 4 weeks and monthly thereafter.
- Daily doses are usually divided and sustained-release preparations are normally given twice daily.
- Dose adjustment may be necessary in diarrhoea, vomiting and heavy sweating.
- To prevent relapse of mania and depression, serum levels of 0.4–1.0 mmol/l should be aimed for.
- For prophylaxis of bipolar depression, the ideal therapeutic range is 0.8–1.0 mmol/l.

Side effects

- Short term:
    diarrhoea
    fine tremor

indigestion
nausea
polydypsia
polyuria
fatigue.

- Long term:
  The above *plus*:
  exacerbation of psoriasis
  hypothyroidism
  memory loss
  weight gain.

Overdosage

- The following *will* occur with severe Li$^+$ overdose, i.e. plasma concentration >2 mmol/l:
  hyper-reflexia
  hyperextension of limbs
  convulsions
  toxic psychoses
  syncope
  oliguria
  circulatory failure
  coma.

- The following *may* occur with severe Li$^+$ overdose:
  goitre
  raised antidiuretic hormone concentration
  hypothyroidism
  hypokalaemia
  ECG changes
  exacerbation of psoriasis
  kidney changes
  death.

Drugs affecting Li+ levels

- Drugs that increase plasma Li$^+$:
  phenylbutazone and possibly other NSAIDs

thiazide diuretics, e.g. bendrofluazide (Aprinox, Centyl, Neo Naclex), chlorthalidone (Hygroton), xipamide (Diurexan) and indapamide (Natrilix)

other K^+-sparing diuretics, e.g. triamterene (Dytac) do not have any effect on serum Li^+

since ibuprofen is available over the counter (OTC), patients should be warned of the possible adverse effects; aspirin has no such effect.

- Drugs that decrease plasma Li^+:
  theophylline
  acetazolamide
  Sandocal
  Fybogel
  some antacids, e.g. sodium bicarbonate, magnesium trisilicate (Gaviscon).

NB Cessation of Li^+ therapy 2–3 days before elective surgery should be considered, although the risk of precipitating a psychotic relapse should be weighed against the benefits.

Investigation of leg ulcers

- Measuring the ankle/arm pressure index (API) with a Doppler probe (often carried out by the district nurse) enables venous ulcers (70% of leg ulcers) to be distinguished from ulcers where impaired arterial perfusion is the likely cause.

- Patients with an API of <0.8 should be referred for arterial assessment.

Interpreting DEXA scans in screening for osteoporosis

- DEXA scanning, most accurate at the hip, is an accurate screening tool for those at risk of osteoporosis:

women who have had an early, natural or surgical menopause
under the age of 45 years

women or men with a previous fragility fracture, height loss
or kyphosis

any patient on more than 7.5 mg of steroids for more than 3
months

patients with secondary causes of osteoporosis, such as hyperparathyroidism, hyper- or hypothyroidism and alcohol abuse.

INTERPRETING DEXA SCAN RESULTS

- The T-score is the comparison with the young adult mean and
  indicates an absolute fracture risk:

  a T-score of > –1.0 is normal

  a T-score of between –1.0 and –2.5 indicates osteopenia and
  advice should be given on diet, weight-bearing exercise,
  smoking (stopping) and calcium and vitamin D supplements, and HRT may be considered

  a T-score of < –2.5 indicates established osteoporosis and may
  require additional treatment.

- The Z-score is the patient's relative risk for their age:

  a Z-score of >1 indicates an increased risk of fracture.

INVESTIGATIONS IN PATIENTS WITH OSTEOPOROSIS BEFORE COMMENCING TREATMENT

- FBC – look at MCV for possible alcohol excess.
- ESR to exclude myeloma.
- LFTs for possible alcohol excess.
- Protein electrophoresis if ESR is raised.
- Calcium, raised >2.65 mmol/l in hypercalcaemia, possibly
  due to hyperparathyroidism (raised parathyroid hormone
  (n=12–72)) or secondary cancer (consider breast and lung).
- Testosterone, SHBG, LH, FSH, low testosterone or free testosterone index with raised gonadotrophins, indicating hyper-
  gonadotrophic hypogonadism; low gonadotrophins indicates
  hypogonadotrophic hypogonadism.
- Endomysial antibodies for coeliac disease (though 20% false
  negative rate).

INDEX